LOVE YOUR CHOLESTEROL

Dr Robert A Buist PhD

Love Your Cholesterol
Copyright © Robert Buist 2014

Integrated Therapies Pty Ltd
PO Box 370
Manly NSW 1655
Australia

Cover Design by Loc Le

ISBN 13: 978-0-9925252-0-0
ISBN 10: 0-9925252-0-9

Contents

Acknowledgements

My wife, Wendy, deserves top credit, because as editor of *International Clinical Nutrition Review* for 22 years, she was the ideal person to meticulously edit, rewrite and methodically transform much of the heavy science into digestible prose. Ultimately, she pulled the entire script into a meaningful shape.

I would also like to thank Dr Mark Houston and Dr Ross Walker who are two cardiologists who were an inspiration for much of my work, particularly Dr Walker for his valued suggestions.

For the colour diagrams and early editing, I would also like to thank Melissa Lee who managed to find the time in her busy schedule to pick up the oversights and add a little colour and pictorial sense to the text.

Mary Cavaggion, from NutriPath Integrative and Functional Pathology Services, was also generous in allowing me to publish some of the Liposcreen LDL subfraction graphs and associated biochemistry in Chapter 6. These are typical of the lipoprotein data from their Cardiovascular Profile testing and give the reader an outline of these new tests for cholesterol.

I would also like to thank Daniel Urbinder and Andrew Whitfieldcook for their support and help in retrieval of reference material that allowed me to move some of these new ideas into the mainstream.

Finally, I would like to thank Julie Spearritt for helping me to navigate through the minefield of online publishing.

About the Author

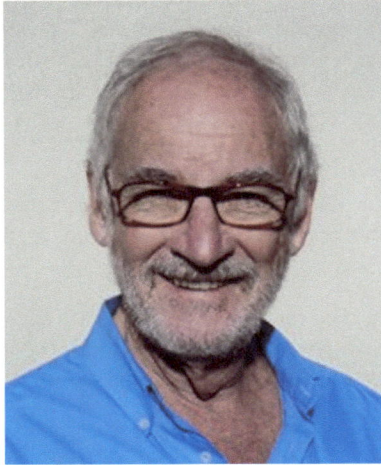

Robert A Buist BSc(hons), PhD

Robert has an honors degree in biochemistry and a PhD in medicinal chemistry and pharmacology.

After 8 years in asthma and cardiovascular drug research at Macquarie University, and later as a Postdoctoral Research Fellow at New York State Health Department, he switched his research focus to the newly emerging field of Nutritional Biochemistry and Complementary Medicine. This change lead to further graduate qualifications in chiropractic and naturopathic medicine. He is presently acknowledged as one of the founders of Nutritional Medicine in Australia.

For 22 years Robert was also Editor-in-Chief of the international quarterly journal, *Clinical Nutrition Review* and is the author of three best-selling books on contemporary nutrition. He is presently part of the Bioceuticals Scientific Advisory Team in Sydney, Australia and is a formulator of nutritional products and functional foods. He lectures widely and has been a regular presenter/guest on radio and TV for over 30 years.

Foreword

For too long, modern society has been given the misconception that cholesterol in food and the bloodstream is an evil killer that clogs arteries. We have been "fed" a similar line regarding saturated fat and cardiovascular disease.

The problem with both these concepts is that they are too simplistic and are fundamentally incorrect. In his new book, Dr Buist explains clearly the widespread misconception regarding this entire subject and presents the solid science behind the correct place for cholesterol and its relation to cardiovascular disease.

This book is required reading for health professionals involved in the care of patients and those at risk for cardiovascular disease but the language and presentation also makes it an informative read for anyone interested in maintaining a healthy cardiovascular system.

Dr Ross Walker MB. BS (hons), FRACP, FCSANZ
Consultant Cardiologist

Introduction

What's not to love about cholesterol? It's not a question you hear very often, despite the fact that cholesterol is critical for life. Without it we would die. How many of us are aware that cholesterol is of paramount importance as a building block for most of the cellular and hormonal functions of the body. Cellular functions, biochemical pathways and hormonal circuits would close down without it. The function of every organ and tissue would be in jeopardy, including the brain, which has a particular attraction for cholesterol and even has specialised cells to manufacture more when needed. Without adequate cholesterol you wouldn't even be attempting to read this book. Even the sunshine that gives life to all animals and plants on the earth relies on cholesterol in our skin to manufacture vitamin D, a vitamin that in turn drives several hundred key biochemical reactions in the body.

Humans have been eating cholesterol-containing animal products for thousands of years. We also make cholesterol inside our bodies. It's time we started to appreciate that cholesterol is one of the most important molecules that we humans both make and need.

So perhaps the real bone of contention does not involve cholesterol levels per se. Other little understood aspects of its production and delivery to tissues are much more informative. While some aspects of human biochemistry have little scope for variability and exist in a well-defined and narrow range in all people (like body temperature, blood pH and serum glucose), the picture is not the same when it comes to cholesterol levels. Each person appears to have a different cholesterol "set point" depending upon hereditary, lifestyle and temporary individual need associated with fluctuating stress and health issues. All evidence indicates that our body, in its wisdom, sets these levels depending on metabolic need by facilitating or blocking the body's manufacture. From an early age people appear to have a set point for cholesterol which can vary from 3mmol/l to 9 mmol/l. These levels may silently resist change for decades, while a person stays in good health.

You might be starting to wonder why cholesterol is so demonized if it serves so many useful functions. Why has cholesterol phobia gripped everyone over the age of 40 in an unyielding vice? We talk about "good" cholesterol and "bad" cholesterol without really knowing what we are trying to define. Cholesterol is just a single chemical entity with a very specific blueprint for manufacture in the body. It is neither good nor bad. Just very necessary. The drive to lower total cholesterol has also become an obsession with most doctors who frequently seem to overlook its critical function in the body.

Protocol for best medical practice is intimately linked to a widespread subservience to the pharmaceutical industry. The research that continues to demand lower and lower levels of cholesterol as the body's natural "set point", is funded by this industry and for the most part it is evaluated by those who are financially dependent on such funding. Conflict of interest is endemic.

So it's very encouraging to see the evolution of a different strand of research that is shedding new light on the situation. You could almost say that the old indicators of blood cholesterol status are being blown out of the water. So here are some challenging new ideas.

- The "total cholesterol" measurement may now be meaningless because the cholesterol carrier components have been redefined.

- One part of the so-called "bad" LDL cholesterol may actually be desirable or even incredibly important because it delivers much-needed biological "spare parts" to any tissue in need.

- Some of the so-called "good" HDL cholesterol may actually be non-functional and even a dangerous inflammation-providing molecule in the bloodstream depending upon a host of largely changeable environmental factors.

- Many dietary and lifestyle factors within our control can impact our cholesterol profile for the better.

So if the total cholesterol, LDL and HDL measurements are meaningless without a more in depth look at the entire cholesterol transport system, it's fair to say that doctors and pathology labs are now acting on an outdated system and data which is inadequate at best, and inaccurate or irrelevant at worst.

This new information surrounding cholesterol carriers explains why clinical studies frequently show that high cholesterol levels are actually advantageous. It also explains why lowering cholesterol with statin drugs may be placing one's general health in a precarious situation for reasons other than the adverse side effects of the statins themselves (and other cholesterol-lowering medication).

In the search for an understanding of the mechanism behind heart disease and arteriosclerosis, cholesterol has been made the scapegoat. But it isn't the cause.

Whatever our natural cholesterol level, almost all of us can learn how to keep it safe and in the best possible shape. Understanding how cholesterol works (things like dietary intake, body synthesis and transport around the body) is the first step. Then with the help of good medical advice and by educating ourselves about the other less well-known side of cholesterol research-the part of the picture linked to lifestyle, diet and natural supplements-we can truly empower ourselves to make whatever changes may be necessary to optimise our cholesterol levels, in most cases without taking drugs. We can truly learn to know and love our cholesterol.

I realise that there is a lot of science in this book and while it may at times seem overwhelming, I believe the degree of is necessary to shed real light on a fundamentally flawed belief system about the nature of cholesterol. Health professionals will appreciate this and these days one should never underestimate the desire of the public for the facts.

Chapter 1: The Cholesterol Studies

At the beginning of the 20th century heart disease was rarely seen. Now it is the biggest killer in the Western world and most people have been led to believe that the culprit is cholesterol.

The Early Cholesterol Trials—Rabbits Were the Wrong Guinea Pigs

Let's look at some of the early research into cholesterol.

Over 50 years ago a young Russian researcher named David Krichevsky decided to carry out experiments to see whether dietary cholesterol was related to a rapid recent increase in heart disease. He chose rabbits as the experimental subjects and fed them 5% by weight of their diet as cholesterol. But rabbits are herbivores. They never eat cholesterol. Cholesterol only comes from an animal source. No vegetable contains cholesterol. Grasses are usually the sole food of rabbits and they certainly don't eat fatty animal foods or cholesterol-laden foods derived from animals. Rabbits are able to make their own fat by a fermentation process, which takes place in their hindgut. (1) (2)

> Only animal foods contain cholesterol. It's ludicrous to see sunflower, corn, soya, safflower and olive oils in supermarkets with "cholesterol free" slashed across the label. Of course they are cholesterol free. They don't come from an animal source. They come from plants.

So rabbits were the wrong model to use to test cholesterol, given that their biochemistry and physiology has not evolved to handle animal foods. Feeding rabbits cholesterol is equivalent to us eating grass, leaves or hay. Our physiology cannot digest or metabolize these foods. We do, however, have the ability to metabolize dietary fats and make cholesterol in our bodies.

It really is important for all species to eat the foods they have evolved to handle. The cow is another good example of an animal designed to digest grass and fibre, not animal products. It has an extra stomach and also has the ability to ferment the cellulose and other indigestible fibres it gets from grass. We are still wondering about the real facts behind Mad Cow Disease, but it appears to have something to do with cows being fed offal from other animals.

At the beginning of the 20th century it had been shown in similar experiments that feeding cholesterol to rabbits resulted in cholesterol accumulation in all tissues, including cirrhosis of the liver, enlarged adrenals and cholesterol deposits at other sites besides the hardened arteries, because the animals did not have the metabolism to handle excessive quantities of cholesterol.

Fudging the Facts? The Seven Countries Study

The myth that dietary cholesterol and saturated fats cause heart disease really took off in the late 1950s when Ancel Keys, an American scientist who studied the influence of diet on health, published a study (The Seven Countries Study), which compared heart disease and fat consumption in seven different countries. For his purposes he chose the US, Finland, the Netherlands, Italy, the former Yugoslavia, Greece and Japan. (3)

The results of the Seven Countries Study suggest that the higher the concentration of fat in the diet, the higher the incidence of heart disease. This has remained one of the key points of "evidence" linking increased cholesterol consumption and coronary heart disease.

However, there was one really glaring problem with this study and it's called "selection bias". This is one of the most perfect illustrations of that handy little trick which occurs when scientists design an experiment to serve their own purposes or to achieve a desired outcome by selecting only certain facts and ignoring others.

Keys had a large range of countries from which to choose his data. Twenty two in all. He left out countries with high fat consumption and very little heart disease. He also left out countries with low fat consumption but a lot of heart disease.

Had Dr Keys chosen some of the other countries in his original study, like Switzerland, Finland, France, Sweden, Israel, the Netherlands and Germany, he would have ended up with the opposite result.

The outcome? Despite selection bias, Keys' efforts gave rise to a theory that is now called the "Lipid Hypothesis" which claims that eating saturated fats will raise your cholesterol and cause heart disease. It's a hypothesis which has been disproved, as you will read in later chapters.

Keys did, however, correctly promote the importance of monounsaturated fat, claiming "all-cause and coronary heart disease death rates were low in cohorts with olive oil as the main fat". On the positive side, Keys is best known for promoting the concept of the Mediterranean diet.

The Truth Starts to Emerge

The large and enormously prestigious Framingham Study started at Harvard University Medical School in 1948 and is still continuing. It gave rise to the original dietary "risk factors" for heart disease with which we are all so familiar today. Six thousand people took part in the study. Those on high cholesterol, high saturated fat diets were compared with those on low cholesterol, low saturated fat diets.

The Framingham researchers thought that they knew exactly why some people had higher cholesterol levels than others. The hypothesis was that these people simply ate more cholesterol in their diet. But did they?

The outcomes... were very interesting, persuasive, but unexpected. After 40 years one of the Framingham directors, William Castelli, commented on the results of the study. He said, "...the more saturated fat one ate, the more cholesterol one ate, the more calories one ate, the lower the person's serum cholesterol...we found that people who ate the most cholesterol, ate the most saturated fat, ate the most calories, weighed the least and were the most physically active." (4)

> People with cholesterol lower than 200 (ie 5.17mmol/l) suffer nearly 40% of all heart attacks". William Castelli

More Evidence Goes Against Expectations

The Multiple Risk Factors Intervention Trial (MRFIT) was another huge multi-centered trial organized to look at the same parameters. Researchers hypothesized that multiple risk factors would be synergistic, and were expecting a "better" outcome in comparison with what was then looked on as a failure with Framingham. (5)

MRFIT involved 28 medical centers, 250 researchers and led to the screening of 361,662 men of whom 12,866 were considered to be at very high risk of heart disease. (6)

The Outcome: After cutting the participants' consumption of cholesterol by 42%, saturated fat by 28% and total calories by 21%, their blood cholesterol dropped only slightly and the incidence of coronary heart disease was unaffected. This made a few people sit up and listen. Here was yet another example of how drastic lowering of dietary cholesterol and saturated fat had no effect on the course of the heart disease.

Population Studies: Embarrassing the Experts?

In future chapters we'll look more into the idea that while food doesn't have much of an effect on cholesterol levels it has a huge effect on the quality of the cholesterol carriers in your body, and whether or not they are likely to do their job properly. We will also look at the role of different dietary fats and oils. Meanwhile it provides a helpful perspective to get an idea of how many people around the world are living heart healthy lives without dietary or medical manipulation. It's also interesting to keep in mind that the health of these populations is declining the more they move away from their traditional diet and bring in the processed "foods" so popular in the west.

Mary Enig and Sally Fallon Morell have correlated some definitive research on the role of saturated fat and cholesterol in human health. (7) On traditional populations they have this to say: "Numerous surveys of traditional populations have yielded information that is an embarrassment to the Diet Dictocrats." It would be difficult to find any of the studies cited below being mentioned by those urging restriction of saturated fats. That's why we want you to read more about them.

So where's the best place to live for heart health and happy cholesterol levels? Consider this research while deciding whether you need to move house or just borrow a certain style of cookbook from the library. One book you shouldn't miss is Fallon and Enig's book, Nourishing Traditions.

France

The French love fatty foods like duck liver pate, butter, cream, eggs and cheese. The essence of the French Paradox is that the French have among the world's highest levels of saturated fat consumption and among the world's lowest levels of heart disease. Gascony, an area of France famous for the production of duck liver pate (foie gras) has a remarkably low level of death from heart disease (80 deaths per 100,000). Compare this with statistics from the United States, where the heart related death rate for middle aged men is 315 per 100,000. (8)

France vs Ireland

Data was taken from the WHO MONICA project. Researchers found cardiovascular disease 3-4 times more common in Belfast than Toulouse. Reasons uncertain. The Irish ate more saturated fat and the French ate more "cholesterol". Seems they couldn't point the finger at anything to do with particular fat consumption patterns as they concluded that "major differences are present for several food items, and in general these differences add support to the antioxidant hypothesis". In particular, the Toulouse sample ate more fruit, vegetables and wine. We'll look more at that particular hypothesis a bit later. Another hint: it may also have something to do with the fact that fats in the context of a healthy antioxidant rich diet, act differently to fats examined in the laboratory. Or maybe the French and Irish have different types of hearts, hence this research paper carries a more alluring title than many: "Autres pays, autres coeurs?" (9)

Mediterranean

Before moving too far from France, let's look around other Mediterranean countries that have low rates of heart disease even though fat-including highly saturated fat from lamb, sausage and goat cheese-can comprise up to 70% of their caloric intake. The inhabitants of Crete, for example, are remarkable for their good health and longevity as are the Italians, Spanish, etc. Olive oil and fish, of course, are high sources of what has been called "good fat". Nuts and even snails play their part. Spanish researchers put the effectiveness of this style of diet down to two main factors, both of which we will explore in more detail in later chapters. But key facts to hold on to for the moment: "on the one hand, the Mediterranean diet increases high-density lipoprotein cholesterol (HDL-c) plasma levels and on the other hand, it decreases the susceptibility of low-density lipoprotein cholesterol (LDL-c) to oxidation. This is why the Mediterranean diet must be recommended in order to prevent heart disease". (10)

Japan

The Japanese diet since the second world war has been high in protein and fat with plenty of beef, pork, eggs, chicken, fish and other seafood and yet they have the longest lifespan of any country. In Okinawa, where the average life span for women is 84 years (even longer than in the rest of Japan), the inhabitants traditionally eat generous amounts of pork and seafood and do all their cooking in lard rather than oil. Sesame oil is used as a garnish.

There is some controversy about what the Okinawans really eat, with well-known scientist, Dr Craig Wilson, promoting a low fat story while others beg to differ. In fact, Okinawa is sometimes known as the Land of Pork and this meat is much loved by the locals. Since Buddhism is not followed on the island, there are no taboos against eating animal foods. Okinawan-based gerontologist, Dr Kazuhiko Tiara, claims that the local diet is "very healthy, and very, very greasy". Meat intake is at least 100g per day, and this doesn't include fish, tofu, eggs, etc. Even though Okinawans have the highest fat and protein intake in Japan, their diet can also be considered vegetable-based. Daily stir-fries of vegetables include the blood sugar-stabilizing bitter lemon. These are fried in lard and generously laced with fatty pork. Okinawans raise much of their pork free range, often on their own land. Pasture-fed pork is as high in monounsaturated oil as olives, as well as being a good source of vitamin D. (11)

> ### What do Okinawans really eat?
>
> "The whole pig is eaten-everything from "tails to nails." Local menus offer boiled pigs feet, entrail soup and shredded ears. Pork is cooked in a mixture of soy sauce, ginger, kelp and small amounts of sugar, then sliced and chopped up for stir fry dishes. Okinawans eat about 100 grams of meat per day-compared to 70 in Japan and just over 20 in China-and at least an equal amount of fish, for a total of about 200 grams per day, compared to 280 grams per person per day of meat and fish in America. Lard-not vegetable oil-is used for cooking.
>
> Okinawans also eat plenty of fibrous root crops such as taro and sweet potatoes. They consume rice and noodles, but not as the main component of the diet. They eat a variety of vegetables such as carrots, white radish, cabbage and greens, both fresh and pickled. Bland tofu is part of the diet, consumed in traditional ways, but on the whole Okinawan cuisine is spicy. Pork dishes are flavoured with a mixture of ginger and brown sugar, with chilli oil and with "the wicked bite of bitter melon".
>
> Deborah Franklyn (12)

Yemenite Jews

Jews living in Yemen with a diet containing fats solely of animal origin experience very little heart disease. On the other hand, Yemenite Jews living in Israel experience high levels of both heart disease and diabetes. The diet eaten in Israel is much higher in vegetable oils and margarine. Refined sugar is also consumed in large amounts in Israel, but very little in Yemen.

India

A comparison of populations in northern and southern India revealed a similar pattern. People in northern India consume 17 times more animal fat but have an incidence of coronary heart disease seven times lower than people in southern India.

Africa

The diet of African tribes like the Masai are comprised largely of milk, blood and beef, yet they don't suffer from heart disease or unhealthy cholesterol levels.

Eskimos

Animal fats from fish and marine animals make up the bulk of the Inuit diet. In summer they take advantage of a brief berry season. Before the introduction of processed foods, Eskimos were virtually free of disease and exceptionally hardy.

China

An extensive study of diet and disease patterns in China found that the region in which the populace consumes large amounts of whole milk had half the rate of heart disease compared to several districts in which only small amounts of animal products are consumed.

Russia

In long living populations in Soviet Georgia it was found that those who eat the most fatty meat, live the longest.

Melanesia

The Kitawa Study showed no existence of heart disease in a population who lived on a fresh tropical diet of fruit and vegetables, plus generous amounts of fish and coconuts. Coconuts are high in saturated fat and this gave the Kitawa population a saturated fat intake similar to Sweden.

Switzerland and Austria

The Swiss brought us fondue. They enjoy remarkable longevity on one of the world's fattiest diets. In neighbouring Austria, the story is very similar.

Greece

It's a similar story. High fat diet, excellent longevity.

The United States

One big dietary experiment, as we have already discussed. A huge reduction in dietary saturated fat intake during the course of the 20th century was not accompanied by a decrease in heart disease. Between 1910 and 1970 there was a general decline in animal fat consumption in the American diet of about 20%. Butter consumption decreased even more. Yet there was in fact an exponential increase in heart disease during the century.

You may ask yourself how this happened if a high level of saturated fat in the diet was a major cause of cardiovascular disease? If you lower the amount of saturated fat in the diet surely the incidence of heart disease must drop. How can you thin out the enemy but your soldiers keep dying at an even greater rate?

Truth of the matter is that saturated fat consumption wasn't the only thing to change. What about the consumption of vegetable oils and sugar? People started consuming vast quantities of margarine, safflower, sunflower, corn, soya, cottonseed and other refined cooking oils. There was a 400% increase in the consumption of these unstable oils accompanied by a 60% increase in the intake of sugar and processed foods. This is a radical change in two major food groups and this is where we should start looking if we want to find the reason for the explosive increase in heart disease over the last century and why today 40% of people in the US die of heart disease each year.

> Between 1910 and 1970 there was a general decline in animal fat consumption in the American diet of about 20%. Butter consumption decreased even more.
>
> Yet there was in fact an exponential increase in heart disease during the century.

The Elderly

The elderly are considered a population in their own right. Please read more about this crucial topic, together with the relevant research, in chapter 3. The essence of the message is that in elderly populations, high cholesterol appears to correlate with greater longevity and lower morbidity. That is, by the time you're 85 high cholesterol is associated with a longer and healthier life.

Chapter 2: Why We Absolutely Need Cholesterol

The body has a mind of its own. Daily it can make 3-4 times more cholesterol than you actually eat. In fact it can make around 1000-3000 mg each day. As we've just mentioned in the introduction, when we are getting very little cholesterol from our food, the body kick-starts its own production. Conversely, when there's plenty of dietary cholesterol the body turns down its own production. Any excess cholesterol that the cells do not need is transported back to the liver where it's converted into bile salts and other fat packages for recycling.

> Cholesterol doesn't exist in a vacuum.
> It's a major metabolic controller.

Let's briefly have a look at just why we need a good supply of cholesterol in the body. Just for the record, cholesterol isn't really a fat at all. It's a steroid and its vital functions include hormone production, cellular, intestinal, nerve, brain, liver, bone health and more. Cholesterol is critical for our survival.

Cell Membranes—Some Facts

- Cholesterol exists in every cell of the body.

- Around 90% of cholesterol is found within cells, not in the blood stream as you might expect.

- Cholesterol prevents the walls of the cell from collapsing into a blubbery heap. It is essential for cell structure. Without adequate cholesterol, cell walls easily lose their rigidity and under the internal pressure of cells can expand outwards, causing bloating of cells, malfunction of their day to day activity and even destruction.

- Our cells are designed with "lipid rafts". Made of protein and cholesterol, these are specific areas of the cell membrane where cholesterol is concentrated. It is the lipid rafts that act as the glue that holds us together and influences the structure, thickness, permeability, and shape-changing ability of cell membranes. Membrane stability depends upon these cholesterol-rich rafts and when cholesterol is depleted the entire action of cell membranes throughout the body is in disarray. The entire structure of the cell membrane depends on cholesterol.

- Cholesterol also affects cell function, that is, it controls the comings and goings of molecules into and out of the cell and keeps cellular communications open. Healthy cell membranes are also vital for letting nutrients and hormones in and out, for protection against toxins entering and for the removal of waste material arising from the normal metabolism of each cell. Lipid rafts also regulate cell migration (movement) and the way in which cells talk to one another and generally control membrane trafficking i.e. the movement of vital ingredients and waste products, both into and out of cells.

- Cholesterol is needed to repair damaged arteries. When arteries are damaged due to multiple attacks by free radicals, oxidized lipids, glycated molecules (where sugar attaches to them), and other toxins, cholesterol is mobilized to the scene of the crime to help in the repair of the arterial lesion.

The Skin—Some Facts

- Skin structure relies on the integrity of the cell membrane and is therefore highly dependent on an available supply of cholesterol.

- Skin is the starting material for the production of vitamin D. Vitamin D3, also known as cholecalciferol, is produced by the skin when it's exposed to ultraviolet B (UVB) radiation. This process is dependent on adequate levels of cholesterol in skin membranes. Healthy bones are also dependent on this system functioning well.

- Cholesterol in the skin helps us to hold water so that we do not dehydrate. The outer layers of the skin need cholesterol to prevent water loss and protect against the sun's harmful rays. Moist, soft, supple skin depends upon having a good supply of cholesterol.

- Protection from external water soluble toxins depends on the integrity and flexibility of skin structure.

Without adequate cholesterol we easily become depleted in the essential fatty acids that keep skin healthy, resulting in problems like:

- Dry, dull skin (e.g., feet/face/general)
- Scaly or flaky skin (e.g., legs)
- Cracking/peeling fingertips & skin (e.g., heels)
- Small bumps on back of upper arms
- Patchy dullness &/or colour variation of skin
- Mixed oily and dry skin ("combination" skin)
- Irregular quilted appearance of skin (e.g., legs)

The Liver—Some Facts

- About 50-60% of the cholesterol made in the body is produced in the liver.

- One of the most important functions of the liver is to make bile acids. These are made from cholesterol and are stored in the bile fluid of the gall bladder and are released into the intestines after eating a fatty meal where they serve the purpose of emulsifying fats in our diet, ready for absorption into the body.

Cholesterol Makes Bile Salts

Bile salts play a critical role in emulsifying all our dietary animal fats and fat soluble nutrients including the hundreds of fat soluble vegetable-derived nutrients called phytonutrients. That's to say, they prepare all fatty or fat soluble plant-derived nutrients in foods like fruits, vegetables, legumes, grains, sprouts, herbs and spices so that the body can absorb them properly.

- Without cholesterol we would not be able to process dietary fats and essential fatty acids (such as omega-3 and omega-6 oils). This would lead to a breakdown in their digestion and absorption capabilities.

- Without cholesterol we couldn't absorb fat-soluble vitamins (such as vitamins A, D, E and K and other fat soluble vegetable-derived nutrients (phytonutrients) such as beta carotene). We would very quickly come down with the symptoms of fat soluble vitamin deficiency and essential fatty acid deficiency.

Signs/Symptoms of Essential Fatty Acid Deficiency include:

- All types of skin problems (see above)
- Thick or cracked calluses
- Dandruff or cradle cap
- Dry, lackluster, brittle or unruly hair
- Soft, fraying, splitting or brittle fingernails
- Dull nails-lack of surface shine
- Slow growing fingernails
- Dry eyes
- Dry mouth/throat
- Inadequate vaginal lubrication
- Menstrual cramps
- Premenstrual breast pain/tenderness
- Excessive ear wax
- Excessive thirst
- Allergies (e.g., eczema/asthma/hay fever/hives)
- Craving for fatty foods
- Stiff or painful joints

The Brain and Nervous System—Some Facts

- The brain represents just 2–3% of your body weight but contains 25% of the body's cholesterol while 60% of the brain's dry weight is fat-cholesterol and fat are of paramount importance to brain function.

Without cholesterol you can't think.

- Lowering cholesterol in the membranes of the brain and central nervous system (CNS) by only 10% can interfere with nerve transmission.

- In the nervous system, all membrane function, synapse formation (synapses are where one nerve passes on information to another nerve and the nerve signal is able to travel) and insulation around the nerves called the myelin sheath are dependent upon cholesterol to function. Cholesterol controls the synapse where neurotransmitters facilitate thoughts and emotions.

- Cognitive problems are the second most reported side effect from taking cholesterol-lowering drugs. Some statin drugs can directly interfere with the local synthesis and availability of cholesterol in vital areas of the brain.

- Cholesterol-lowering drugs such as lovastatin and simvastatin penetrate the brain and central nervous system (CNS). Simvastatin is a statin drug which can easily cross the blood brain barrier (whereas pravastatin can't). This means that simvastatin can then badly affect the creation and maintenance of structures relevant to memory.

- Unlike other parts of the body, the CNS only produces enough cholesterol to survive and it draws on extra cells when it needs to create extra nerve junctions and to expand and repair networks. So important is cholesterol for the brain's functioning that there are special nerve cells called glia that manufacture cholesterol on site.

- In an analysis of 324 emails from people taking statins 30% reported mood changes such as depression, irritability, and anxiety. (1)

It is uncertain to what extent the cognitive losses related to statin usage can be reversed by discontinuing the drugs. They will certainly reoccur with further administration.

Low Cholesterol Affects Mood and Behaviour—Some Facts

- *When your cholesterol level changes, so does your mood and mental health.* This is a new finding worth highlighting.

German researchers observed 65 adult inpatients in a university psychiatric hospital. Major depressive symptoms were found to coexist with low levels of LDL and HDL but the LDL/HDL ratio in these depressed patients was much higher than usual. What's most interesting about this study is that patients in remission from their depression also spontaneously changed their LDL/HDL ratio to a less atherogenic composition and their HDL (good cholesterol) levels rose. (2)

- Low serum cholesterol has now been linked in many scientific papers with accidents, suicide, aggressive behaviour, impulsive acts, hostility, depression and antisocial personality. Cholesterol lowering treatments with statins have demonstrated an association between non-illness related mortality from suicides, accidents and violence. A correlation has been suggested between depression and cholesterol-lowering drugs.

- When patients who complained about statin side effects were asked survey questions, 65% of 843 spoke of increased anxiety or irritability and 32% reported an increase in depressive symptoms. (3)

- In clinical practice, severe anger and irritability have been observed in some statin users.

Studies Linking Low Cholesterol with Suicidal Behaviour

- French study: In 6393 working men aged 43-52, both low serum cholesterol and declining cholesterols were associated with increased risk of death from suicide. (4)

- Israeli study: Similar results were obtained from 584 psychiatric patients. Patients who had attempted suicide had significantly lower serum cholesterol than non-suicidal patients. (5)

- US Study: Payne Whitney Psychiatric Clinic in New York Hospital. Male psychiatric patients with the lowest cholesterol levels were twice as likely to commit suicide compared to those with the highest levels. (6)

- Human and animal research indicates that low or lowered cholesterol levels may reduce serotonin activity. This affects mood, appetite, sleep, memory and learning.

- An excess of violent deaths in men without prior heart disease who were randomly assigned to low cholesterol diets has been observed in some meta-analyses of randomized trials.

Serotonin and Violence

In 1998 Dr Beatrice Golomb reviewed all existing studies on low cholesterol and violence. Some take-home facts include:

- Human and animal research, indicate that low or lowered cholesterol levels may reduce serotonin activity.

- Serotonin is a neurotransmitter in the brain that regulates mood, appetite, and sleep.

- Serotonin's cognitive functions include memory and learning.

- Modulation of serotonin at synapses is one of the major actions of several classes of antidepressant drugs.

- Animals with low serotonin activity are more likely to be aggressive. (7)

- Antisocial behaviour has been linked with low cholesterol. Of 274 subjects with personality disorders, the 139 with antisocial personality had lower cholesterol levels than the group with other personality disorders. (8)

Other Studies Linking Low Cholesterol Level and Depression

Finnish research

National Public Health Institute, 29,133 men aged 50-69 years followed up for 5-8 years. Blood samples were analyzed for cholesterol concentrations. Self-reported depression, data on hospital treatments due to depressive disorders from records from the National Hospital Discharge Register and deaths from suicide were measured.

Results showed that serum total cholesterol was associated with low mood and subsequently a heightened risk of hospital treatment due to major depressive disorder and of death from suicide. (9)

French research

In men 65 years and older, low levels of LDL cholesterol (the so called "risk factor"), was actually associated with an increased risk of depression.

In women 65 and older, low levels of HDL cholesterol (the so called "good" cholesterol" was associated with an increased risk of depression. (10)

American research

Among men 70 years and older, depression was three times more common in the group with low plasma cholesterol (<4.14mmol/l). (11)

Balancing Steroid Metabolism—Some Facts

- Cholesterol is the building block for steroids.
- Steroids are involved with blood pressure control and protecting the body under chronic stress.
- The major hormones synthesised by the adrenal glands use cholesterol as the starting material.
- Adrenal gland deficiency patients with low levels of cortisol (the major chronic stress hormone) frequently suffer from low blood pressure and hypoglycaemia.
- Chronic degenerative diseases would flourish if we were to lower cortisol and vitamin D levels.

Diagram 1: Steroid Hormone Synthesis

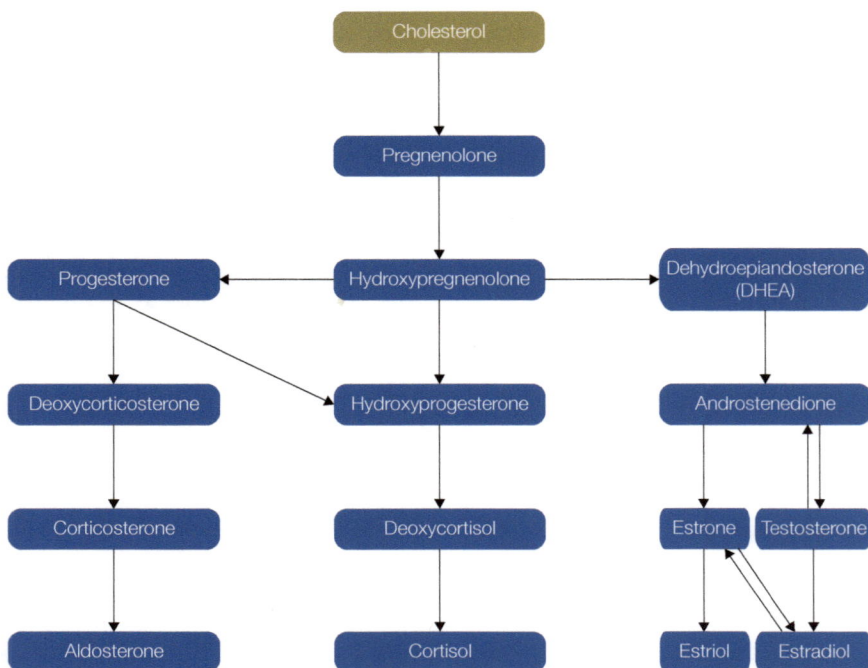

- Excessive urination and dehydration can occur when the adrenal glands don't produce enough of a hormone called aldosterone. Without cholesterol at a reasonable level the body can't make mineralocorticoids like aldosterone. Aldosterone deficiency can cause low sodium and high potassium levels in the blood. This makes the kidneys unable to concentrate urine. This results in excessive urination that can lead to dehydration.

- Our ability to deal with stress depends on steroids produced from cholesterol. Without cholesterol at a reasonable level the body can't make glucocorticoids. The primary corticosteroid is cortisol, made from cholesterol. It is our major stress hormone and swings into action when we are under chronic stress. It stimulates the breakdown of fat and protein to release fatty acids and amino acids, which go on to produce glucose when we need it. In this way cortisol is overseeing the production of extra macronutrients to supply additional energy to see us through a difficult stressful period.

Together with adrenaline (epinephrine) it increases blood glucose in response to stressful situations by inhibiting its uptake into muscle and fat cells. It strengthens contractions of the heart muscle. It increases water retention and has anti-inflammatory and anti-allergic effects. Cortisol plays a role in the body's sensitivity to insulin and helps maintain healthy cardiovascular function, blood pressure, inflammatory responses and metabolism.

Cholesterol is the building block for all of our sex hormones like oestrogen, progesterone and testosterone. All androgens, oestrogens and progesterone are made using cholesterol as the starting material (See Diagram 1).Testosterone is one of our major androgens. It is responsible for our sex drive. It enhances muscle mass, cell growth and secondary sex characteristics. DHEA (Dehydroepiandrosterone) is the primary precursor of natural oestrogens such as oestradiol and is manufactured from cholesterol. (12)

Can you imagine what would happen if we couldn't get enough cholesterol to manufacture these important hormones?

Coping with Stress—Some Facts and Alternative Hypotheses

Elevated cholesterol levels may not be a cause of blocked arteries and heart disease. As we have just seen, cholesterol is the building block for the manufacture of our major chronic stress hormone, cortisol. It has been suggested that rather than blocking arteries cholesterol may be performing another function. Cortisol is elevated when a person enters a period of their life that entails chronic stress. Alpha-male middle aged executives-ambitious, building careers, striving for success-are extremely prone to heart attack. However high cholesterol, rather than attacking arteries, may simply be a marker of increased stress levels and an inadequate lifestyle including poor diet and lack of exercise, and it is these factors that lead to the heart attack.

The Adrenaline/Cortisol/Cholesterol Connection

During stressful periods (fright, fight, flight) adrenaline can be released in large amounts leading to constriction of blood vessels and blood clots as it mobilises sugar, fatty acids and more cholesterol into the bloodstream.

High cholesterol is associated with both high adrenaline levels and high blood cortisol.

- The body protects us from physical stress and trauma by releasing chemicals known as "acute phase reactants" with less well-known names which include C-reactive protein, complement, interferon, fibrinogen, ferritin, ceruloplasmin and amyloid. These molecules protect us when there is inflammation, blood loss, trauma, fatigue and the need for healing.

- Humans have not evolved and adapted to produce hormones suited to the different types of mental and emotional stressors found in modern society. The daily stressors now involve new and different fears. Anxieties can include failing to keep up with changing technology, worries about losing jobs in a time of financial instability, financing a home purchase or a long retirement or vulnerability in the face of ageism. Such things now drive our hormones and neurotransmitters and lead to a different kind of stress.

A Total Change in the Nature of Stress

No longer do we have to worry about escaping a wild beast or catching one if we are to enjoy a good meal. We now have a world of canned foods, refrigerators, handy supermarkets and a predictable system of law to protect us.

Different factors now drive our hormones and neurotransmitters and lead to a different kind of stress. Our old fright, fight and flight stress network is just a little redundant. This structure that served us so well in the past to survive physical stressors, is still there and often acts like a hair trigger but it is usually without any real present physical cause. We no longer need to increase our clotting tendency, we don't need to replace iron due to rapid blood loss, we don't need to accelerate healing of tissue and we don't need to increase blood flow into a traumatized area by growing new blood vessels.

The agitation, exhaustion, anger, irrationality and a host of other feelings which now dominate and often consume our lives when the stress mechanism is in action, can find no traction. The consequences of these are heart disease, diabetes, obesity, metabolic syndrome and other diseases caused by stress related disorders of metabolism. Remember, chronic stress leads to excessive cortisol release. This leads to rapid conversion of muscle protein to sugar.

Healthy people can release more growth hormone during this situation to help conserve muscle protein. People who eat sugar to excess are unable to do this. The result is suppression of growth hormone release and a loss of muscle protein. Cortisol increases protein release, which increases blood sugar, which increases insulin, which converts the extra sugar to fat and drives the whole obesity scenario.

This is a major factor in the present increased incidence of age-related metabolic syndrome and is linked to the obesity epidemic. After the age of 40 years there is a tendency to lose muscles and convert them into fat. This is called sarcopaenia and this accelerates with age and is a chronic problem for 45% of people over the age of 65 years. Those with the most muscle burn fat most efficiently.

Ironically, those same people who were genetically equipped to cope best thousands of years ago due to very efficient responses to stressful situations (i.e. quickly releasing stress hormones when physically threatened) are now very likely the same genetic group that responds to chronic mental stress in an exaggerated way, potentially leading to or exacerbating heart disease, obesity, diabetes and other indicators of metabolic syndrome.

Without adequate cholesterol we would cease to absorb the essential nutrients for optimal function and survival. Bones would deteriorate and digestive function would start to break down. Stress levels would rise to an unimaginable level and all sexual activity would cease. Muscle complaints, cognitive problems and memory loss would be rife. The list goes on. Could this possibly be happening already in our statin-dominated world?

Chapter 3: Longevity—Cholesterol and the Elderly

Key Point

- In elderly people, higher cholesterol is often associated with better cardiovascular health and longer life.

People aged 80 years or older are the fastest growing population in high-income countries. In this age group lipid-lowering treatment is common, especially in the US, UK and Australia. Most European countries are more reluctant to get on the band wagon of prescribing cholesterol-lowering drugs to older people, although it's been reported that one-third of Swedes aged 75-84 are now treated with statins. (1)

According to the Green Health watchdog, pharmaceutical companies who manufacture drugs for cholesterol management see the over 65s as a "particularly lucrative market sector". Why wouldn't they? By 2040 the over 65s will represent the purchasing power of around 300 million people. Advances will no doubt run parallel in the growing area of neuromarketing. It will not be hard to tap the fear of heart disease and stoke in this elderly group. The push towards over-the-counter sale of statin drugs has already achieved success in the UK and is unlikely to be far away in the US. Now if your elderly British bus driver is worried about his cholesterol he can self medicate. It's not necessarily good for his driving. Remember this when you read the chapter on the side effects of statins. (2)

Yet even back when my first cholesterol book, *The Cholesterol Myth*, was published in 1992, the indications were all there that higher cholesterol per se was no problem for the elderly, and may in fact be linked to longer life and better health. Has anything new come up? Were we ill-informed back then?

The answer is no. Confirmation of these hypotheses has continued to occur, although you wouldn't necessarily think so due to the universal blitz that continues to cast "cholesterol" as public enemy #1. The idea that high cholesterol is a risk factor at the highest ages seems to be based on an assumption that research on younger adults is relevant to the elderly. This is not the case.

> People older than 85 years of age are protected by high cholesterol.
>
> The data show that each 1mmol/l increase in total cholesterol corresponded to a 15% DECREASE in mortality.

The fact is that in older populations higher cholesterol has been shown to be protective. What's more, low cholesterol may be one of the major risk factors in heart attacks, heart failure and ischaemic stroke as well as a range of other serious health problems and all-cause mortality. It's the older people with high cholesterol who are likely to live longer and are especially protected against cardiovascular problems, cancer and lethal infections causing hospitalizations.

Over the last 35 years I have had numerous conversations with colleagues and friends discussing the implications of growing old on cardiovascular health.

A typical conversation might go something like this one with a 62 year old friend of mine. "My GP said that my cholesterol was up. It was 6.2 mmol/l but it's been like that for years. He seems worried that I am about to have a heart attack or stroke and wants me to go on statin drugs but I'm feeling great. What should I do?".

I usually explain that having a cholesterol of 6.2 mmol/l isn't dangerous per se, and may in fact be protective for anyone over 60 years of age. This is particularly so if the lipoprotein carriers of cholesterol have not been damaged.

I suggest such people stop worrying. The statistics are actually working in their favour, although that doesn't mean no effort is required. Embracing all the suggestions in this book will go a long way towards keeping your cholesterol carriers (the lipoproteins) in the best possible shape.

In later chapters we'll discuss in detail ways to address the potential problems associated with damaged liporoteins carriers in the bloodstream such as oxidized LDL, glycation and the lack of antioxidants and the importance of the size of LDL and HDL and their number.

So I do suggest to my older friends and colleagues that they give serious thought to embarking on a cholesterol-lowering regime with statin medications. There is plenty of evidence suggesting that they may do more harm than good. There are alternative approaches to diagnosis and treatment.

Let's look at some of the research that has come out since my original book went to press. Some of the studies have been conducted specifically on groups of women, but as you will read, high cholesterol appears to be protective across gender.

Yale University

In 997 subjects 70 years of age or over, high levels of total serum cholesterol, or low levels of the "good" HDL cholesterol, were not associated with a significantly higher rate of all-cause mortality, coronary heart disease mortality, hospitalization for myocardial infarction or unstable angina. (3)

Lancet publication

724 research subjects, average age 89 years, were divided into 3 cholesterol groups:

(a) cholesterols of <5.00 mmol/l

(b) 5.0-6.4 mmol/l

(c) >or equal to 6.5mmol/l.

Not surprisingly in such an elderly sample during 10 years of follow-up 642 people across all cholesterol groups died and the main cause of death was cardiovascular disease. What's interesting is that the data showed that each 1mmol/l increase in total cholesterol corresponded to a 15% decrease in mortality.

What's more, mortality from cancer and infection was significantly lower among the participants in the highest total cholesterol category than in the other categories, which largely explained the lower all-cause mortality in this category. (4)

The 2001 Honolulu Heart Study

3,741 men aged 51 to 73 years. Blood was taken in 1971 and again in 1991.

Highest death rate was associated with those who had the lowest cholesterol level on both occasions. The authors concluded, "These data cast doubt on the scientific justification for lowering cholesterol to very low concentrations in elderly people." (5)

A Review of Observational Studies in the Elderly

Total cholesterol lower than 5.5 mmol/l was associated with the highest mortality rate in the 80+ group.

All-cause mortality was highest when total cholesterol (TC) was lowest ('a reverse J-shaped' association between TC and all-cause mortality). (6)

Elderly Women, Cholesterol and Mortality

Nursing home, 92 women, free from cancer, followed-up for 5 years. During this period 53 died and only one had cancer.

Mortality was lowest at a serum cholesterol of 7.0mmol/l. Mortality was 5.2 times higher at the lower cholesterol level of 4.0 mmol/l.

Even at the high cholesterol level of 8.8mmol/l mortality was only 1.8 times higher.

The relation between low cholesterol values and increased mortality was independent of the incidence of cancer. (7)

> Female and over 60? You may be interested to know that your risk of dying is much higher when you have low rather than high cholesterol.

A huge 15 year follow-up study of 149,650 men and women showed that in men, across the entire age range, although of borderline significance under the age of 50, and in women from the age of 50 onward only, *low cholesterol was significantly associated with all-cause mortality, showing significant associations with death through cancer, liver diseases, and mental diseases.* For the first time, this study demonstrated the dangers of low cholesterol and that it occurred even among younger respondents, contradicting the previous assessments among groups of older people that this is a proxy or marker for frailty occurring with age. (8)

Random sample of 2277 elderly residents of northern Manhattan (age range 65-98 years), non-demented Medicare recipients, mostly women (66%) and of mixed ethnicity (30% white, 31% black, 38% Hispanic). Subjects followed up for an average of three years, evaluated at 18 month intervals. Thorough original assessment: each patient underwent blood testing, a health interview, assessment of functional capacity, medical history, physical and neurological examination, and a neuropsychological evaluation. National death index used to determine each patient's vital status.

After an average of three years of follow-up, 291 patients had died and it was found that the patients with the lowest total cholesterol and lowest LDL cholesterol were almost twice as likely to die as those with the highest cholesterol levels. (9)

In-Hospital Patients, Cholesterol and Mortality study published in the *American Journal of Medicine*

Subjects were 6984 patients aged 65 years or older who had been admitted to 81 participating medical centers during four survey periods between 1993 and 1998. Patients were divided into four groups based on total cholesterol levels at hospital admission:

<4.14 mmol/l (n = 2115), 4.14 to 5.16mmol/l (n = 2210), 5.16 to 6.2mmol/l (n = 1719), and ?6.2mmol/l (n = 940).

A total of 202 patients died during their hospitalization. *Again the highest mortality was among those with the lowest cholesterol.* The death rate for those with the lowest cholesterol (< 4.14 mmol/l) was 5.2%. At higher cholesterol levels the death rate dropped. Cholesterol levels 4.1-5.16mmol/l (2.2%), 5.16-6.2mmol/l (1.6%) and greater than 6.2 (1.7%). In other words, compared to those with the lowest cholesterol readings, the group with the highest cholesterols had one third the chance of dying.

The researchers concluded, "Among older hospitalized adults, low serum cholesterol levels appear to be an independent predictor of short-term mortality". (10)

Reading through these studies you may have noticed that all-cause mortality is associated with having low cholesterol. This isn't surprising. Let's remember the importance of having adequate cholesterol for every organ and for every vital function in the body—for the skin, liver, adrenals, brain, nervous system, immune system and all the related hormones, bile salts, vitamin D and their association with infections, cancer, liver disease, heart failure and neurological health.

> The concerted drive to rid the body of cholesterol no matter what the consequences persists. Has the unique and universal need for cholesterol in the body been overlooked by doctors, researchers and those making and advocating lipid-lowering drugs?

We are, after all, mortal. One day our heart will stop beating. A cardiovascular event is the most common form of death in the healthy elderly. Such a death is not a failure on anyone's part nor is there a magic pill to prevent it.

Chapter 4: Dangers of Artificially Lowering Cholesterol

The Main Questions

- Will lowering cholesterol stop me having a heart attack?
- Is it possible to manage my cholesterol levels without taking medication?
- Can trying to prevent a heart attack inadvertently lead to heart failure?

In the heart business, there's such a thing as "usual care". No one talks about it much. As you'd expect it's about weight management, quitting cigarettes, healthy diet and regular exercise.

Expensive trials (e.g. ALLHAT-LLT and PROSPER) have found virtually no difference in the outcomes from managing cholesterol with diet or drugs. The research team of Dr David Jenkins, professor of nutritional sciences at the University of Toronto, found that in terms of lowering "bad" LDL cholesterol, statins were 30.9% effective and diet came a close second at 28.6%. It's a broad generalization, based on an imperfect diet, but you get the idea. (1)

Early Drugs Fail to Prevent Cholesterol Absorption

Aimed at lowering cholesterol by preventing absorption from the gut, early drugs such as cholestyramine and clofibrate failed. At the time it was not understood that if you prevent cholesterol absorption from the diet using such drugs, the body simply ramped up its own production. We know that most cholesterol is manufactured by the body itself and that blood cholesterol doesn't rise because of an increase in dietary cholesterol.

This also explains why low cholesterol diets only reduce cholesterol measurements by a few percentage points. There are still quite a number of margarine-type foods which contain phytosterols and other natural cholesterol inhibitors aimed at preventing cholesterol absorption but this doesn't get away from the fact that the body can override these processes by making its own cholesterol.

Consequently, the statin drugs of choice nowadays do not even try to prevent absorption of cholesterol from the gut but rather inhibit the biochemical mechanism that allows the body to manage its own cholesterol level. Such drugs are now ubiquitous, and constitute a multi billion dollar industry. They are also surrounded by a web of controversy.

Dangers of Cholesterol-Lowering Drugs (and Statin Side Effects)

The most commonly prescribed drugs that lower cholesterol these days are known to most of us as "statins". Statins inhibit the body's production of cholesterol by blocking one of the first steps in the biochemical pathway leading to its manufacture. The blocking site is at an enzyme (called HMG Co A reductase) which controls the production of cholesterol in the body and has profound ramifications for every biochemical reaction that uses cholesterol.

The whole issue of side effects comes down to one simple fact: if a drug is blocking your entire cholesterol manufacture and you can't get enough from the diet, you've got problems. If there is a shortfall, dietary cholesterol can only make up for about 10% of it. As we have already pointed out, the brain alone contains 25% cholesterol. No wonder cholesterol-lowering has been associated with problems related to cognition, thinking, memory, behaviour, anxiety, depression etc.

Be Aware—The Most Common Side Effects of Statins

There is a wide range of possibilities when it comes to experiencing side effects from statins, though many are never attributed to the drug in question. The most common is muscle pain or weakness, which can sometimes take an extreme form in what is called rhabdomyolosis (muscle meltdown). Other common side effects are fatigue, memory and cognitive sleep problems and neuropathy. The website of the Mayo clinic provides its own list of side effects. One Californian MD adds a few of his own, including chronic psoriatic rash, lupus-like skin lesions, early Alzheimer's and non-healing deep infections. Others consider that the possibility of statins increasing the risk of various cancers (skin, breast, etc.) is strong.

Side effects can range from mild to debilitating. In the case of pravastatin, for example, 2-7% may experience muscle pain (myalgia), nausea, vomiting, common cold, flu, headache, diarrhoea, skin rash, constipation, fatigue, gas, indigestion or heartburn and 1-2% may experience pain (including stomach, joint and chest), dizziness, liver dysfunction, peripheral neuropathy, muscle cramps and vision problems.

Rhabdomyolosis—Muscle Pain can be Deadly

As we have already pointed out, the major side effect of statins is muscle pain which may be experienced as soreness, tiredness or weakness in the muscles. The pain may be mild or severe enough to interfere with walking, climbing stairs and other general daily physical activities. In rare cases muscle damage can be life-threatening. We call this rhabdomyolosis and it involves the rapid breakdown of skeletal muscle due to injury to the tissue. As well as severe muscle pain, it can result in liver damage, kidney failure, life-long disability and even death.

In 2001 one statin, cerivastatin, was withdrawn from the market because it was found to cause rhabdomyolysis that was 6-12 times greater than with other statins and responsible for 385 non-fatal cases and 52 deaths.

The risk of rhabdomyolosis increases dramatically when statins are taken together with another popular lipid-lowering agent, fibrates. The incidence rises from 3,500:1 to 1,600:1 and for older patients with diabetes 500:1 on the combined therapy. Other factors which can exacerbate the rhabdomyolosis induced by the combined therapy include old age, female gender, kidney or liver disease, hypothyroidism, debilitated status, surgery, trauma, excessive alcohol intake and heavy exercise.

So when it comes to muscle pain, all the statins have been shown to produce muscle disorders in susceptible patients, and muscle pain is one of the most common reasons for patients being taken off statin drugs. One study co-authored by Beatrice Golomb, MD, PhD, director of UC San Diego's Statin Study group, identified nearly 900 studies which mentioned the adverse effects of statins. Dr Golomb found that: "muscle problems are the best known of statin drugs' adverse side effects, but cognitive problems and peripheral neuropathy, or pain or numbness in the extremities like fingers and toes, are also widely reported." (2)

Thousands of cases of *memory dysfunction* have also been reported to the FDA's Medwatch program after people took the statin, Lipitor, but after several years, the agency still hasn't acted. Many people have experienced severe memory loss while on Lipitor. But patients are reluctant to report amnesia, or they attribute the symptoms to old age or early Alzheimer's.

Statins can also exhibit dangerous interactions with other medications and some foods. Grapefruit, for example, contains a substance that can make statins more potent. Also beware of combining statins with some antibiotics, antifungals, antidepressants and immunosuppressant medications.

High dose statins are now in vogue. Levels have been increasing significantly in recent years. So what has been the clinical outcome of this changed strategy? Basically that lowered incidence of heart-related events is more than offset by "death from other causes". What's more these observations fail to take into account the increased incidence of haemorrhagic stroke in those taking high dose statins. This is definitely a "side effect" that needs serious consideration.

Take a look at some of the relevant research into the effects of prescribing "maximum Lipitor":

- The actual outcome was that for every 100 patients with elevated cholesterol levels who take statins for 5 years, a heart attack will be prevented in 1 or 2 patients. However, the maximum dose Lipitor increased the risk of deaths from non-cardiovascular causes. (3)

- Treating New Targets (TNT) study:
  In 2005, 10,001 people with stable heart disease were administered either the Maximum Dose 80mg Lipitor (atorvastatin) or a standard 10mg. Both dosage levels reduced LDL cholesterol but the high dose was more effective. Over 5 years of taking the high dose, 434 people (8.7%) in the high dose group experienced another cardiovascular incident such as a heart attack or stroke compared to 548 people (10.9%) in the 10mg group. This was an improvement of 2.2%. However, this improvement in deaths from cardiovascular causes was completely offset by an increase in deaths from other causes. (4)

- In a study involving 4,731 people who had experienced a recent stroke, maximum dose Lipitor was given to 2,365 people and a placebo given to the other 2,366. While there was a minimal improvement in the high dose Lipitor group of 1.9% reduction in frequency of second stroke compared to placebo, there was also a 67% increase in haemorragic strokes in the high dose group. The high dose Lipitor did not reduce the number of deaths overall. (5)

- Data from a recent meta-analysis of 11 trials including 65,229 people with 244,000 person-years of follow-up in healthy (normal cholesterol levels) but otherwise high-risk men and women showed no *reduction in mortality when treated with statins.* (6)

> The maximum dose Lipitor increased the risk of deaths from non-cardiovascular causes.

"Risk factors", as we discussed earlier, are unreliable predictors for future heart events. Yet the world of medical research is coming up with new ones all the time, and the number currently stands at around 400. Just about everyone will fit the picture somewhere, and this is why so many statin prescriptions are written for people without existing heart disease. Given such formidable side-effects it makes you wonder whether statins should be even considered as prophylactic treatment for otherwise healthy individuals. How would you interpret this data?

Man-Made Deficiency: The Mitochondria and CoQ10

Mitochondria are the little furnaces inside our cells that produce 80% of our food-derived energy. The majority of the energy we get from eating carbohydrates, protein and fat comes from the digestion of our food breakdown products in the mitochondria.

Like a high revving engine there is much activity in these little powerhouses and as a result this is also the place where we produce most of the toxic free radicals in the body, especially if we overeat and put an extra load on this machinery.

When we overeat, all the food is still absorbed and finds its way through the bloodstream to the mitochondria. However the extra load creates such a strain on the biochemical processes that it causes electron leakage as the food components are converted into energy, carbon dioxide and water. This process generates electrons and free radicals, harmful substances which have a destructive effect on the body. When added to the additional intake of free radicals from our polluted external environment, these free radicals make up a toxic army that requires an equal force of antioxidants to control them. So what happens if our mitochondrial function is impaired? The body produces less energy and more "free radicals".

Central to the process of making energy and blocking free radicals is a key chemical compound known as Coenzyme Q10 (CoQ10). It's also called ubiquinone or ubiquinol.

If the little furnaces inside our cells are not working properly (impaired mitochondria) we produce *more free radicals than we can handle*. This is where CoQ10 comes into its own.

The big problem is that all statins lower CoQ10 levels. This is because the biochemical pathway that produces cholesterol also produces CoQ10. If you lower one, you lower the other. Statins also reduce the blood carriers that transport CoQ10 and other fat-soluble antioxidants to important tissues of the body. And we're not just talking about some small effect. Studies have found that statins can lower CoQ10 serum levels by 40%. Cellular levels could be reduced even more. (7) (8) This situation creates real problems for the heart.

The Statin, CoEnzyme Q10 and Heart Failure Loop

CoEnzyme Q10 ensures that the heart muscle has sufficient energy and when levels drop there is an increased possibility of heart failure. The heart uses up huge quantities of CoQ10.

Few people realize that the incidence of congestive heart failure dramatically increased soon after the first statins hit the market, and has been rising ever since. Heart "failure" is not heart attack or stroke. Basically it describes a heart whose muscle (the heart is a muscle) is running out of energy. This form of cardiovascular side effect is largely ignored by most monitors. It appears that the depletion of CoQ10 in the muscles is responsible for more than just the experience of sore skeletal muscles and in fact strongly influences heart function.

What's more, the drug companies appear to know this. In 1989, Merck & Co. Inc. filed two patents for the use of CoQ10 with statins in order to prevent CoQ10 depletion and attendant side effects. The patent applications, which can be viewed online at the United States Patent and Trademark Office website, clearly show that the statin manufacturer was aware of the link between CoQ10 depletion and heart failure. But to my knowledge this patent has not yet been applied.

Even the Framingham Study mentioned earlier found that low serum levels of CoQ10 were a risk factor for the development of heart failure (HF).

> Biopsies have confirmed that the severity of heart failure correlates with the lowest levels of CoQ10.

Getting a Second Opinion

If you still find it hard to come to grips with the side effects of the statins and in particular, the link to CoQ10, try imagining you are one of the patients of Dr Peter Langsjoen, cardiologist, as reported in the journal, Biofactors, in 2005. He found that 50 consecutive new patients reported one or more side effects from statin therapy. In response, the statin drugs were discontinued and CoQ10 therapy was instigated instead. Patients were followed for an average of 28 months and the following observations on the prevalence of side effects noted.

The high prevalence of skeletal muscle pain and weakness at 64% on initial visit was reduced to 6% at follow-up.

Fatigue decreased from 84% to 16%.

Shortness of breath went from 58% down to 12%.

Memory loss was reduced from 8% to 4% .

Peripheral neuropathy decreased from 10% to 2%.

There were no adverse effects from ceasing the drug therapy, just an improvement in heart function when the drugs stopped and the coenzyme Q10 was started.

Please talk to a qualified health practitioner if you are personally concerned about the side effects of any drug. (9)

Man-made Heart Failure

Take a moment to read through a few more relevant studies linking low cholesterol to the risk of heart failure. The results are surprising, counterintuitive, or unwelcome, depending on where you're coming from. In this brief wrap up of the research you will no doubt come across lots of information which hasn't hit the headlines on TV, the internet or in the newspapers. This is important news, yet has received little attention.

In 1998 it was first reported that lower levels of total cholesterol, low-density lipoprotein (LDL), high-density lipoprotein (HDL), and triglycerides were predictors of higher mortality in 222 patients with advanced heart failure. *Lower total cholesterol was the single best predictor of death* among 16 variables. (10)

In 2003 Rauchhaus and coworkers reported in the Journal of the American College of Cardiology the results of a study involving 114 chronic heart failure patients. They found that *a total cholesterol level <5.17mmol/l (200 mg/dl) predicted a poor clinical outcome independently of other risk factors.* (11)

Briefly, the study investigated the relationship between cholesterol levels and all-cause mortality in chronic heart failure (CHF) in a group of 114 patients with moderate to severe heart failure (the derivation study) and then applied the results to a second group of 303 unselected patients with mild to moderate CHF (called the validation study).

In the first study, survival at one year was 78% and at three years was 56%. Increasing total serum cholesterol was found to be a predictor of survival independent of the cause of CHF, age, force of the heart beat, and exercise capacity, with a 36% increase in the risk of death within three years for every mmol/L *decrease* in serum cholesterol. In the validation population, one-year survival was 88% and three-year survival was 68%. The chance of survival increased 25% for each mmol/L of increased increment in total cholesterol.

No-one's really game to say it but this research does raise the possibility that statins may be dangerous in these patients. One of this research team, Dr Andrew Clark from the University of Hull (UK), had this to say: *"In heart failure, the fatter you are and the higher your cholesterol, the better off you will be. My recommendation at the moment is not to use statins in heart failure patients. I have no evidence to believe that they are good and quite a lot of suspicious evidence that they are bad."*

In 2003 in the same journal Fonarow and Horwich also reported a relationship between cholesterol, lipoproteins, and mortality in 1,134 patients with advanced heart failure arising from multiple causes. This study found that low total cholesterol levels were associated with characteristics known to predict worse outcomes in heart failure. Low total cholesterol was also associated with more severe symptoms of heart failure. Low total cholesterol was a strong, independent predictor of increased mortality in this group. Patients with higher LDL, HDL, and triglyceride levels also had significantly longer survival. Fewer than 25% of the patients with the lowest cholesterol (<3.34mmol/l; 129 mg/dl) survived at five years, whereas survival was >50% for patients with the highest cholesterol (>or= 4.9mmol/l; 190 mg/dl). This study clearly established that higher levels of total cholesterol and lipoproteins were associated with improved long term survival in patients with heart failure, confirming the findings of the smaller, shorter term studies. (12)

How can we explain these results? The researchers themselves note that *heart failure is a metabolically stressful illness. In this light, a high cholesterol level might be seen as beneficial, as it indicates a greater reserve to deal with metabolic stress.* They also note that molecules that carry cholesterol through the blood stream (lipoproteins), may have a specific protective role in heart failure.

What's more, they point out that cholesterol-carrying lipoproteins are good at absorbing bacterial endotoxin (a toxin associated with the bacterial cell wall). Immune system activation occurs in heart failure patients because of weakness in the bowel wall (oedema), allowing bacteria to transfer into the body. It may be that lipoproteins carry out a beneficial role by mopping up any bacterial proteins before they cause immune system activation.

Even though we can't be 100% sure of cause and effect, the researchers do suggest that lower cholesterol levels can now provide a valid, independent risk prediction for mortality in patients with chronic heart failure. The facts can't be ignored: "heart failure patients with total cholesterol levels of below 4.9-5.2mmol/l (190 to 200 mg/dL) are at 1.5 to 3 times the risk of dying compared with those with higher levels of total cholesterol".

So you're getting the idea about the negative link between low cholesterol, statin use and heart failure. Unfortunately people with heart failure are not invited to take part in scientific studies that might shed light on this problem. It's not buying into a conspiracy theory to suggest that scientific studies are put together in ways that will make side effects appear minimal, or ideally disappear. All major statin trials aim to eliminate class III and IV (advanced) heart failure patients, and *it's generally true to say that cholesterol-lowering drugs are not tested on people with cardiovascular risk. That would be unethical.*

In fact when pharmaceutical companies publish adverse side effects of statins they tend to divide major categories of side effects into 6 or 7 different categories in order to keep the scarier ones under 1%. For example, Joel M. Kauffman, PhD, research professor of chemistry and biochemistry at the University of the Sciences in Philadelphia said that amnesia could be divided into confusion, memory loss, senility, and cognitive impairment. This is one method by which a major watershed of side effects can be turned into a series of streamlets. When they are not all added together the statistics don't look nearly as bad.

It's interesting to note that within two months of the 2003 Fonarow/Horwich study linking cholesterol with heart failure, the same authors published another paper essentially recanting any suggestion that statin use may be implicated in this problem. (13) Let's just say the jury is still out on that one. While there may still be no way of making definitive conclusions regarding the management of individuals with heart disease in general and heart failure in particular, the thoughts of the Rauchhaus group are worth taking on board: *The balance of risk attributable to cholesterol favors high levels in patients with chronic heart failure, even with an ischemic etiology.* (14)

Chapter 5: Inflammation—Global Warming on an Individual Scale

---

Key Points

- Inflammation is a major factor causing heart disease.
- C-reactive protein is one important way we can measure inflammation.
- There are natural ways to decrease inflammation.
- Obesity-induced inflammation accelerates blood vessel disease.

With so many side effects you may wonder why statins are still being used. It's true that we're finally starting to realize that the cholesterol level has seemingly little to do with cardiovascular disease. So is there a better approach?

An obvious reason this question doesn't get asked is that the drug companies are doing very well financially with statins and have an incentive to leave things as they are. However we can also look at statins in a rather different way. It now appears that the degree to which statins work is probably not particularly related to cholesterol-lowering activity, but as the result of an inherent and previously unsuspected, anti-inflammatory action.

Research papers are now being published on the anti-inflammatory and immunomodulatory properties of statins. Inflammation suppression is becoming the new goal. That's good, but *it's important to note right up front that there are other ways of reducing inflammation which are more natural and virtually free of side effects.*

The Role of Inflammation

What do we mean by inflammation? It's one of nature's most basic defenses against injury, trauma and damage to tissue. This damage to tissue may be caused by anything from a stabbing or an abrasive wound, a burn, or an invasion by infectious microbes or chemicals. The body mobilizes everything at hand-the immune and clotting mechanisms, the blood-forming and lymph systems, the liver, and many others. It also mobilizes cholesterol. The inflammatory process is critical to our survival, but it can get out of hand.

Understanding Plaque

Our arteries are a good example of where the inflammatory process can cause destruction. Damage to the lining of the blood vessels can be caused by mechanical stress, tobacco smoke, foreign chemicals, heavy metals and microbial agents (such as helicobacter pylori, chlamydia pneumoniae, toxic periodontal bacteria in your mouth and herpes simplex). Similar problems can be caused by high levels of homocysteine, iron/copper overload, trans fatty acids, oxidized cholesterol and fatty acids (such as linoleic acid hydroperoxide) and glycation due to excess sugars.

Atherosclerotic plaque is formed in an attempt to heal these local injuries. It works like this. Special white blood cells (macrophages) engulf destructive substances, but they ultimately become part of the plaque that clogs arteries. These are known as "foam cells". In its final stages, inflammation associated with these foam cells stimulates the production of new capillaries and connective tissue cells, and induces scar formation. In the case of cardiovascular disease this inflammatory process culminates in plaque formation (Diagram 2).

Scientists were actually exposed to the idea that there might be a link between cell damage and plaque formation over 100 years ago. In 1911 Klotz and Manning published their findings in the *Journal of Pathology and Bacteriology*. (1) They claimed that plaques are the result of local degeneration of the blood vessel wall caused by microbial infection or some other toxic presence. In short, caused by inflammation.

In 1976 Ross and Glomset offered their hypothesis in the *New England Journal of Medicine*, that atherosclerosis is an inflammatory process and a response-to-injury where initiation is a localized injury to the inner wall of the arteries. Atherosclerotic plaques are formed in an attempt to heal these local injuries to the lining of arterial walls. (2)

Diagram 2: How Plaque Forms

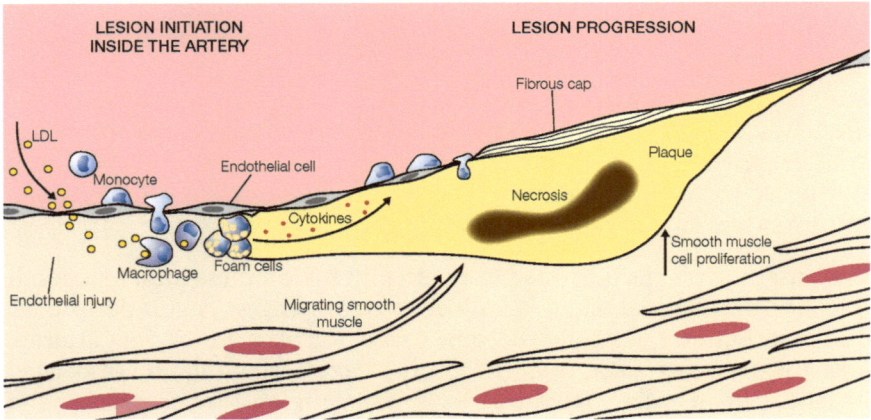

Detecting Inflammation in the Blood

Over the last 15 years hundreds of studies and research papers have been published on the subject of inflammation and cardiovascular disease. An obvious question is whether it's now possible to detect this inflammation in our bloodstream at an early stage in order to prevent the hardening of arteries due to the build up of plaque. The best we are doing at the moment is measuring levels of C-reactive protein.

Whenever inflammation arises in the body the liver produces a marker called C-reactive protein (CRP). This marker is elevated by all kinds of inflammation including burns, trauma, infections, inflammatory arthritis and certain cancers.

The elevation of CRP has also been linked to atherosclerosis and heart disease. In this case a more highly sensitive measurement is used, termed hsCRP. However, this test is still not particularly accurate and may be influenced by infections or inflammation in other parts of the body. Any readings must be analyzed in association with all other known risk factors such as smoking, diabetes, high blood pressure, obesity etc.

Cardiovascular Risk /CRP levels

- Low risk for cardiovascular disease if CRP is 1 mg/l or less

- Moderate risk for cardiovascular disease if CRP is between 1 and 3 mg/l

- High risk for cardiovascular disease if CRP greater than 3 mg/l

- A CRP level greater than 10 mg/l may be seen in an acute plaque rupture such as, a heart attack or stroke, provided there is no other explanation for the elevated level (other inflammatory or infectious process).
  The American Heart Association (AHA) and the Centre for Disease Control (CDC) (3)

Cholesterol Repairs Inflamed Vessels

When a building becomes dilapidated and needs repair, with any luck it will soon be swarming with carpenters, brick layers, tilers, plasterers and painters. At a cursory glance one may think that this sudden influx of people is responsible for the damage done to the house rather than working on its repair. We may now view high blood cholesterol in the same way.

Whenever we need to make more tissue, heal wounds or repair tissue, as is the case when there is inflammation in an artery wall, we need more cholesterol on hand to do the job. You will remember that cholesterol constitutes a huge percentage of the structure of cells and cell membranes.

High cholesterol has come to be associated with hardened arteries and arteries containing plaque, but the crux of the matter is that cholesterol is being used in the repair process. *It is part of the solution not the problem.*

Statins and Inflammation

Statins were produced to inhibit the production of cholesterol. This was a mistake although one that the relevant parties find hard to admit. Statins' main claim to fame should have been their anti-inflammatory action. With the state of our present knowledge about statins' adverse side effects, we should now be turning our research focus to more natural anti-inflammatory agents which don't have the adverse effects of statins.

Obesity as an Inflammation Issue

Obesity is closely associated with both cardiovascular health and chronic low-grade inflammation. Both the fat tissue and the associated macrophages attracted to the fat tissue produce inflammation-provoking substances (like interleukins and TNF-alpha) while the liver responds by pumping out C-reactive protein (CRP) and other facilitators of inflammation.

Solving our personal problems with weight management, let alone the obesity epidemic, is easier said than done. Many factors are involved and each is a huge challenge: genetics, the changes in our food supply, chemicals in the environment, the amount of food being consumed, lack of digestive capacity and unhealthy gut flora, chronic stress, sedentary lifestyle. The list goes on. We have tried to cover many of these factors elsewhere in the book.

Much work has been done over the last 30 years on the value of under eating, or at least cutting back on habitual amounts consumed. In the research world this is referred to as "calorie restriction" (CR). Whether you lean personally towards a high protein diet or one based on unrefined carbohydrates, it appears that the type of food consumed matters less than the quantity, as long as food is of good quality and unrefined. Simply cutting back will slow the production of oxidized fats and free radicals, which are associated with all kinds of degenerative diseases.

Starvation diets, however, don't work. Nutritionally unbalanced diets don't work and fad diets don't work. If we starve ourselves the body's homeostasis mechanisms reset themselves to conserve energy. Many people have gone on the latest diet fad and found that after 6 months or a year that they are back to where they started, if not even heavier because their body responded to the dietary change by going into overdrive and conserving energy. Weight gain was the result of this "body reset" in metabolism.

The key point here is that obesity-induced inflammation accelerates blood vessel damage. Elevated levels of CRP have been tied in with the earliest arterial changes, eventually leading to hardening of the arteries. Chronic subclinical inflammation has been associated causally with insulin resistance (a precursor to diabetes) and metabolic syndrome. Central obesity that first appears in childhood is a strong predictor of metabolic syndrome. So it's important to make the changes and it is possible. (4)

The Importance of Calorie Restriction

Let's take just one research example. A group from the Department of Internal Medicine, Washington University School of Medicine evaluated the effects of calorie restriction (CR) on risk factors for atherosclerosis in individuals who were restricting food intake to slow ageing. They compared 18 individuals who had been on CR for an average of 6 years with 18 age-matched healthy individuals on typical American diets. (5)

The results were quite profound and demonstrated what an incredible impact just lowering your calorie intake can have on all parameters of health. The improvements in the calorie restriction group were not only better; in most cases they were significantly better. After an average of six years the following findings were published:

- the CR group weighed 20% less
- in the CR group body fat was 8.7% compared to the typical American diet group which had 24%
- serum total cholesterol was lower in the CR group
- LDL cholesterol was lower in the CR group
- the ratio of total cholesterol to HDL was lower in the CR group
- triglycerides were lower in the CR group
- fasting blood glucose was lower in the CR group
- fasting insulin was lower in the CR group
- C reactive protein was lower in the CR group
- platelet derived growth factor was lower in the CR group
- systolic and diastolic blood pressure were lower in the CR group
- protective HDL was higher in the CR group
- thickening in the carotid artery (an artery that feeds the brain) was 40% less in the CR group.

Consider the huge amount of money poured into drugs designed to lower cholesterol, control blood sugar, reduce blood pressure etc. with imperfect results and notable side effects. By simply cutting down on what we eat each day and monitoring the quality of our food, we can get the same or better result with the most noticeable side effect being an improved sense of health and wellbeing.

For most people it can be as simple as using a smaller dinner plate and not going for second helpings. Eat at the table, eat slowly and chew your food well. This can make a big difference.

At the time of writing I find many of my patients are doing well on a form of calorie restriction known as intermittent fasting. One such regime, made popular by medical journalist, Dr Michael Mosley, is known as the Fast Diet. (6) Two days a week you limit calories and eat light. It seems to be a simple and effective option for many.

Factors You Can Control

- Don't overeat—control portion size.

- Introduce "light eating days"—fresh food, fewer calories.

- Choose fresh, natural food.

- Eat a rainbow of colourful vegetables and fruit every day.

- Maximize antioxidant intake with seasonal fruits and vegetables plus liberal use of herbs and spices.

- Educate yourself about healthy fats and oils, as healthy fats are essential.

- Avoid the "white devils"—sugar and refined carbohydrates.

- Eat adequate amounts of good quality protein favoring seafood, lean meat, legumes, whey protein.

- Eat more consciously and slowly. Taste your food and chew. Enjoy relaxed company at a table and avoid using mealtimes for arguments and high adrenalin conversation.

Chapter 6: Changing Ideas of "Good" and "Bad" Cholesterol

So far we have highlighted some salient points about cholesterol:

- Cholesterol is a major metabolic controller critical for our very survival.

- A drastic lowering of dietary cholesterol and saturated fat has little or no effect on the course of heart disease.

- The older we get the more dependent we become on having higher levels of cholesterol for optimal health and longevity.

- Cholesterol-lowering statin drugs are frequently counterproductive and have a high incidence of adverse effects.

What else do we need to know? Basically our whole understanding of the cholesterol issue needs an overhaul. We'll now examine some other important issues like these:

- Our previous understanding of "good" and "bad" cholesterol is outdated and inaccurate.

- You can also mess up your LDL cholesterol with sugar, stress and the wrong fats and oils.

- Different cholesterol carriers are neither good nor bad. They simply have different functions.

- LDL is "bad" when it's damaged. The red light is flashing these days for "oxidized cholesterol" (oxidized and glycated LDL). A diet high in processed food predisposes us to cholesterol and fatty acid damage.

- LDL is also dangerous when its shape is "small and dense" and the numbers are high, but healthy when it's "large and fluffy".

- Polyunsaturated vegetable oils, which easily go rancid, are best avoided.

- Good levels of dietary antioxidants help avoid LDL damage.

- New, more detailed tests are becoming available which will give us much more information about the state and function of our lipoproteins-the cholesterol carriers.

What are Lipoproteins

To understand cholesterol we firstly need to understand lipoproteins. Lipoproteins are a variety of complex carrier molecules. All fats that enter our gastrointestinal (GI) tract via the food we eat are packaged in the intestine firstly into lipoproteins called chylomicrons which then regroup into VLDL (very low density lipoproteins) which contain the highest concentration of triglycerides. These are then converted into LDL (low density lipoprotein) the so-called cardiovascular risk factor which takes cholesterol and other fats into the tissues of the body.

As you can see from the Diagram 3 below, LDL is composed of cholesterol, phospholipids, antioxidants and a protein called apoB-100 in the outer layer as well as cholesterol esters and triglycerides in the inner section.

Diagram 3: The Composition of LDL

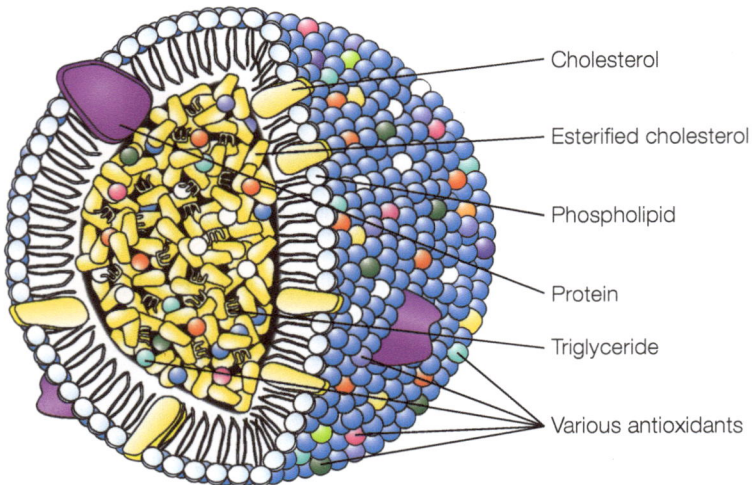

Finally HDL (high density lipoprotein) is a different lipoprotein which takes excess cholesterol from the walls of our blood vessels back to the liver for reprocessing. This is why HDL is called "good cholesterol".

"High cholesterol is among the risk factors for heart disease, but is not the leading risk factor. The most prevalent risk factor is low HDL, along with small LDL particles. In fact, of every 100 people with coronary heart disease, 60-70 will have low HDL and small LDL particles, but fewer than 30 will have high LDL." (1)

So what's really going on with the smaller sized LDL-the real "bad" cholesterol? Firstly, the greater their number, the worse the situation (see Diagram 4). Secondly they have a larger surface area, which allows them to oxidize more easily. Thirdly, they are more easily "glycated". Glycation (or sugar-coating if you like) is the toxic time bomb we want to avoid. Finally, their small size means they can more easily penetrate the blood vessel wall where they are quickly packed off into "foam" cells which cause fatty plaque. LDL of the larger fluffy variety is not a risk factor for heart disease and the difference can now be determined by tests outlined at the end of this chapter.

Diagram 4: The Smaller the Particle Size, The Greater the Risk

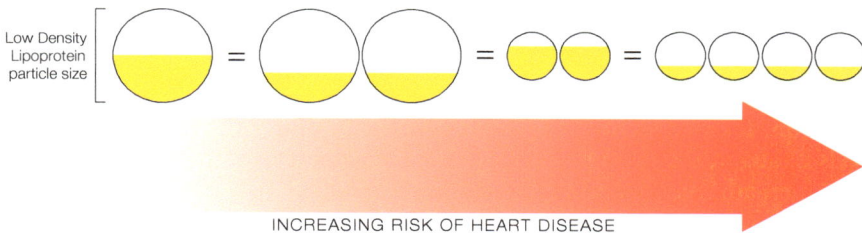

Low Density Lipoprotein particle size

INCREASING RISK OF HEART DISEASE

> The presence of small, dense LDL particles was associated with more than a three-fold increase in coronary heart disease. (2)

When Fat Turns Bad—Oxidized LDL in Heart Disease

Key Points

- A junk food diet predisposes us to damaged lipoproteins and oxidized fat.

- Good levels of dietary antioxidants help avoid LDL becoming oxidized, i.e. going rancid.

- You can also mess up your LDL with sugar, stress and the wrong types of fats and oils.

The higher the concentration of free cholesterol on the surface of the LDL particle, the less vulnerable the LDL particle is to oxidation. By contrast, the higher the concentration of cholesterol that is linked to fatty acids, called "cholesterol esters," (see Diagram 3) the more vulnerable the LDL is to oxidation. This is so because the esters are more likely to be composed of unstable polyunsaturated fatty acids like those found on the supermarket shelves. These fatty acid easily oxidize. Cholesterol esters primarily exist in the core of the particle. The small dense LDL is cholesterol depleted and damaged.

Even if the LDL is not oxidized when it arrives at its destination in the blood vessels, it is still capable of being oxidized when it contacts certain damaged cells that line the blood vessels. This occurs if the LDL package does not have sufficient antioxidant nutrients like vitamin E and CoQ10 in the outer layer to protect it.

Another way of looking at this is to imagine the fat in the LDL as "rancid". Such rancidity indicates that the normal free cholesterol level in the surface layer and the protective antioxidant nutrients are missing or in short supply. It is then called "oxidized" LDL.

Furthermore, it's not only these damaged blood vessel cells that cause such oxidation. It can also occur in the bloodstream under the influence of high levels of sugar, oxidized polyunsaturated vegetable oils, trans fats, free iron or copper, adrenaline and processed "junk food".

Protection with Dietary Antioxidants

A deficiency of antioxidant phytonutrients will also predispose to oxidation. Dietary antioxidants are LDL protectors. They include vitamin E, coenzyme Q10, vitamin C, carotenoids and flavonoids including anthocyanins (the red/blue/purple pigments found in berries and beetroot).

In fact the predominant antioxidant in LDL is vitamin E. After a few years in the medical wilderness it's now becoming much better understood and is known to be a complex of 8 different molecules, tocopherols and tocotrienols, with an average of 6 molecules in each LDL particle.

Other substances with potential antioxidant activity found in the LDL package include beta-carotene, alpha-carotene, lycopene, cryptoxanthin, cantaxanthin, flavonoids such as anthocyanin, phytofluene and ubiquinol-10 (CoQ10). Each is present in amounts of only 1/20th to 1/300th of that of the tocopherols and possibly the tocotrienols. This means that the antioxidant protection of LDL is not overwhelming but it also means that the package is very vulnerable to even slight variations in the oxidative stress level in the blood stream. (3)

It's easy to see how a junk food diet or one high in refined flours, sugar and fat might be lacking in these antioxidant/anti-inflammatory micronutrients, leaving the LDL packages nearly devoid of these protective substances. Antioxidant status may also be lowered when a person is suffering from nutrient-depleting disorders that involve the release of huge quantities of free radicals. This is the case for chronic degenerative diseases and when a person is under chronic stress.

The Role of Lipoprotein (a)

Here's another interesting piece to the jigsaw. Oxidized LDL may also possess an extra piece of protein called apolipoprotein (a) wrapped around the outer layer. This new lipoprotein is called lipoprotein (a) or Lp(a). This is not to be confused with the usual apolipoprotein B-100. What we do know is that virtually all LDL packages containing oxidized phospholipids in the outer shell contain Lp(a). It is now viewed as a strong independent risk factor for atherosclerosis and a marker for LDL oxidation and is found in arterial plaque. The optimum laboratory level of Lp(a) should be under 20mg/dl and preferably under 14mg/dl.

If the LDL is oxidized and has Lp(a) on board, the actual part of the LDL that oxidises is the central core of cholesterol esters and the outer layer of phospholipids. Both of these are composed of the unstable polyunsaturated fatty acids (PUFAs). Bad news. But the good news is that levels of Lp(a) can be reduced with supplemental Coenzyme Q10.

Other nutrients that have been shown to reduce Lp(a) include vitamin C, L-lysine and L-proline. This is because they are vital components for repairing collagen which lines the arteries and can easily become damaged. Collagen must be repaired if wear and tear, ageing and free radicals causes damage to it. (4)

A 28 day randomised, double blind placebo controlled trial was carried out involving 50 patients with acute coronary disease who had a diagnosis of either myocardial infarction (heart attack) or angina and who also had moderately elevated levels of lipoprotein(a). Coenzyme Q10 120mg daily reduced the Lp(a) levels 31% while increasing the protective HDL. LDL and blood glucose also showed a significant reduction in the Coenzyme Q10 group compared to the controls. (5)

The Change from Saturated to Polyunsaturated Food Oils

> **Grandma's kitchen**
>
> *Instructions:*
>
> Take one baked dinner, pour the excess animal fat or lard into a container and keep it at the back of the stove. Use lard for cooking whenever fat is needed.
>
> Surprisingly to the modern mind, after many months this accumulation of saturated fat was still OK. It didn't go rancid despite sitting there at the back of the stove at room temperature and exposed to the oxygen in the air. But it's a totally different story with the present array of vegetable oils (PUFAs).

Where our grandmothers used to cook in lard, dripping and butter, we are now cooking in corn oil, sunflower oil, safflower oil and soya oil. We're told that's a good thing.

Over the last 50 years the balance of dietary fats has changed across the planet as a whole. Polyunsaturated oils (PUFAs) are now the predominant oil in our diet. PUFAs are now plentiful and cheap as witnessed by the huge increase in seed oils in the supermarkets around the world. They are the oils we humans cook with almost exclusively. They are in salad dressings. They are used by the food industry. In India, for example, where the traditional cooking fat in the north is ghee (clarified butter), a saturated fat with excellent stability, the manufacturers (looking for a bigger profit) have now diluted pure ghee with cheap oils.

These PUFAs are VERY unstable. They oxidize easily when exposed to oxygen, light and heat. They are usually so refined that virtually none of the antioxidants that were associated with the original seed are retained. When we buy 1-2 litre plastic containers of these polyunsaturated oils, they are invariably highly processed. They are then frequently heated during cooking, including frying or baking at high temperatures. They may sit around at room temperature in full light for many weeks both before and after opening. Even before we consume these oils they may already be oxidized. This is especially true in the case of commercial fried food such as various forms of "nuggets" and fish and chips where vats of oil are working all day long.

These are also the oils that end up in our fat cells (lipoproteins) and they now predominate in VLDL, LDL and HDL. Is it entirely unexpected that these changes in oil consumption patterns may be having unknown and possibly dire consequences on our health? We have drastically changed what we've been doing for thousands of years. It seems reckless to disregard this food wisdom.

So did the move from saturated fats to polyunsaturated fats have anything to do with the increase in heart disease? You aren't the first to ask. It's a good question.

Rancid Vegetable Oils—Environmental Factors

Short of processing your own olives through an olive press, or crushing sunflower or safflower seeds through a seed press, it's not easy to avoid rancid vegetable oils. We know that there's a high likelihood that the fats and oils we buy are already oxidized long before they get into our bloodstream. But let's suppose for a moment that the oil is cold pressed, contains plenty of oil-protecting antioxidants and is not heated during the food preparation.

Unfortunately we still have a problem. Trying not to put too bleak a slant on it, the problem lies with the widespread oxidative stress levels across the modern environment-with our nutrient depleted, over-refined foods, the polluted air, water and soils. Today there is an exponential increase in oxidative degeneration occurring in many parts of the human body leading to our epidemic of chronic illnesses.

Food that would historically have contained protective antioxidant/anti-inflammatory micronutrients are missing from most diets. Processed foods basically don't contain them. In this situation the unprotected lipoproteins are easily attacked by toxins in the blood stream and become oxidized before they even arrive at the LDL receptor.

The oxidation state of LDL before it is taken up by the cells in the blood vessel wall has been found to be predominantly small, dense LDL which has a higher ratio of oxidized-to-reduced CoQ10 and a lower CoQ10-to-vitamin E ratio. Since CoQ10 is the first line of defence against LDL oxidation, this strongly suggests that oxidation of the small, dense LDL starts earlier than we previously thought.

Oxidized LDL Stimulates Plaque Formation

So now we are looking at a high probability that the LDL in many people is oxidized before it even gets to the blood vessel wall. As we have already noted, oxidized LDL is denser, smaller in size and more dangerous. An interesting case-control study published in the Journal of the American Medical Association in 1988 found that people with small, dense LDL were three times more likely to suffer from a heart attack. The smaller and denser the particles become, and the greater their number, the greater is the chance they will oxidize. They have a greater surface area and are more prone to attack. (6)

When oxidized LDL arrives near the LDL receptor in the blood vessel wall, there are immune cells called macrophages, which can spot trouble. They recognize that the lipoprotein components have been modified by oxidation. Oxidized LDL looks different to these specialized immune surveillance cells. These macrophages use special scavenger receptors to detect the modified or oxidized LDL. They are then taken up into the macrophage and converted into "foam" cells. Foam cells contain the oxidized fat that makes up the plaque which lines the blood vessels at the beginning of the process that causes hardening of the arteries.

An Interesting Anecdote

A cardiovascular surgeon once told a colleague of mine that when he cut through a plaque-laden artery during bypass surgery he noticed a rancid smell associated with the exposed plaque. This fits in with the oxidized lipid story and truly highlights the need for the special macrophages that line the artery ready to pounce on the unsuspecting oxidized LDL packages.

The molecules in the oxidized LDL package that trigger recognition of the LDL damage are predominantly oxidized derivatives of linoleic acid such as linoleic acid hydroperoxide.

Most people probably haven't heard of linoleic acid but it usually makes up around 60% of the polyunsaturated fatty acid content in the vegetable oils found in supermarkets. It's very unstable. *This means that 60% of the cooking oils used in homes today is potentially unstable.*

Saturated fats do not have so many chemically unstable atoms and this is why you can store saturated fats without it going rancid. Similarly saturated fat does not oxidize so easily in the body.

In a 2004 study from Brigham and Women's Hospital and Harvard School of Public Health of postmenopausal women, it was found that the more PUFA they ate, and to a much lesser extent the more carbohydrate they ate, the worse their atherosclerosis became over time. The more saturated fat they ate, the less their atherosclerosis progressed. In the highest intake of saturated fat, atherosclerosis appeared to reverse over time. (7)

It can't be emphasized enough that normal unoxidized LDL is ushered straight into the middle of the cell via the LDL receptor where the cholesterol and other fatty acids are extracted out and used in normal cell metabolism.

Only the modified or oxidized LDL is whisked away by macrophages to become foam cells.

Inflammation and Unstable Plaque

Key Point

- Oxidized LDL causes inflammation. Inflammation leads to the formation of unstable plaque. Unstable plaque is dangerous.

It's the oxidized (damaged) LDL that initiates the inflammatory process involved with atherosclerosis. So what's the mechanism?

Damaged LDL induces foam cells to secrete molecules that attract T cells and other inflammatory cells. It also stimulates the process whereby T cells, foam cells, smooth muscle cells and endothelial cells decrease collagen production and increase collagen degradation. This leads to the rupture of the fibrous plaque. *UNSTABLE plaque is dangerous.*

Plaque disruptions may vary greatly from tiny fissures or erosions of the plaque surface to deep tears involving the surface of the blood vessel which extend into the soft lipid core of the lesion. In all instances some degree of thrombus (clot) formation occurs. In other words, unstable plaque leads to clots which, in the brain, can result in a stroke. In one of the coronary arteries, this can result in a heart attack.

The other negative aspect of oxidized LDL is that it impairs the natural ability of the arteries to produce nitric oxide. Nitric oxide is a natural blood vessel dilator that helps increase blood flow in the vessel. It also decreases blood clotting and helps prevent the oxidation of LDL in the first place.

What about HDL?

Key Points

- HDL is considered "good" because it takes cholesterol away from the arteries. It recycles used cholesterol back to the liver.

- Medical research is moving away from the idea of lowering total and LDL cholesterol and moving more towards the manipulation of HDL. Even the statin researchers are now looking for statins that raise HDL not just reduce LDL.

- Not all HDL is "good". Some doesn't function properly and is pro-inflammatory.

HDL has been called "good" cholesterol because it moves used cholesterol out of the arteries. HDL was thought to be the valuable garbage collector for used cholesterol. Now we know it is just part of cholesterol recycling to other lipoproteins and parts of the body where it's needed.

Initially most attention was focused on lowering total cholesterol and LDL levels but that's now changed . Many researchers agree: "Clinicians have probably been too focused on LDL reduction. However, this approach is no longer justified in view of the documented difference between statins in terms of raising HDL levels, and the trial-based evidence showing the clinically relevant benefits derived from increasing HDL concentrations." (8)

The fact that increasing levels of HDL may be more important in the prevention of heart attack and stroke than reducing the level of LDL, has given rise to some interesting research.

For example, in a 5 year observational study involving 30,067 individuals with type 2 diabetes, results showed that a 6.5mg/dl or greater *decrease* in HDL cholesterol was associated with an 11% increase in cardiovascular disease risk. A 6.5mg/dl increase in HDL cholesterol was associated with an 8% risk reduction.

The authors conclude by saying, "… our results add to the growing body of evidence that increasing the HDL cholesterol levels might be an important strategy for CVD risk reduction. The prevention of HDL cholesterol decreases could be equally important". (9)

In humans each increase in baseline HDL cholesterol of 1mg per deciliter (0.03mmol/liter) is associated with a 6% DECREASE in the risk of death from coronary disease or of myocardial infarction. (10)

How HDL Works

Normally cholesterol can be removed from cells and packed into HDL particles for transfer back to the liver for recycling into VLDL (triglyceride-rich packages) or released into bile as unchanged cholesterol or newly converted bile acids.

The importance of HDL comes into sharp focus when we consider the metabolic imbalance that occurs in cardiovascular disorders such as metabolic syndrome and diabetes, where stored fat tissue releases its fatty acids into the bloodstream (via the liver). This leads to an increase in packages of triglyceride-rich VLDL which can't be broken down as easily due to the lack of specific enzymes in the blood.

The result is a build up of triglycerides, decreased delivery of cell cholesterol to HDL and a subsequent decrease in blood concentration of HDL.

The other problem is that even though HDL has the job of removing cholesterol from the blood (called "reverse cholesterol transport') not all HDL is effective. If one of the protein components of the HDL called apolipoprotein A-1 (apo A-1) becomes damaged by the oxidative mechanism previously mentioned, it becomes useless. Like the damaged small LDL packages, the smaller HDLs are the ones with the damaged apoA-1. They have high levels of pro-oxidant molecules and few antioxidants. The larger HDLs are the effective lipoproteins. They have what is called an effective "cholesterol efflux capacity" and can readily remove cholesterol from the blood vessels to other parts of the body. When the body experiences increased oxidative changes or inflammatory processes, especially in the face of low dietary levels of anti-inflammatory nutrients and antioxidants, the effective HDL can be changed from anti-inflammatory and protective to pro-inflammatory, atherogenic, small and harmful HDLs.

So you can see that the actual level of HDL in the blood does not tell us whether it is effective and functional. We need to measure the size and number of the HDL particles.

A Hypothesis to Watch Out For: HDL and Cholesterol Efflux Capacity

---

Key Points

- Some types of HDL are better at removing cholesterol than others.

- Cholesterol efflux capacity measures HDL *FUNCTION*, not just HDL levels.

Recent research has shown that even though HDL levels may be high this doesn't necessarily mean that there is a reduced risk of coronary heart disease. This risk is reduced only when the HDL has an increased ability to remove cholesterol from the blood vessel wall, especially from the oxidized cholesterol-laden macrophages that are part of the plaque build-up. This may depend on an associated protein that is being looked at presently.

Researchers are now talking about "cholesterol efflux capacity." This is a measure of HDL function.

One such group was Dr Daniel Rader and colleagues at University of Pennsylvania University who published their findings in the January 13th 2011 issue of the *New England Journal of Medicine*. (11) They showed that the cholesterol efflux capacity in 203 healthy volunteers who underwent assessment for hardening of the carotid artery in the neck, 442 patients with confirmed coronary artery disease, and in 351 patients without such confirmed disease, was related to whether or not the person was likely to have coronary artery disease.

They showed that *cholesterol efflux capacity not HDL cholesterol level was the parameter that decided who was more prone to heart disease.*

Additionally, men and current smokers had decreased efflux capacity.

Other Functions of HDL

A variety of other functions of HDL have been described, primarily based on in vitro studies, including anti-inflammatory, anti-oxidant, anti-thrombotic (preventing clot formation), and nitric oxide-inducing mechanisms (keeping the blood vessels open).

One recent study found that *the antioxidant function of HDL is significantly reduced in obese patients compared with healthy controls.* (12)

When people decrease the amount of fat in their diet they usually increase their carbohydrates. *As carbohydrate consumption increases (especially refined carbohydrates and high GI sugars), HDL cholesterol levels decrease and the small dense LDL levels rise.*

Latest Testing for Lipoprotein Fractions

Australian readers may like to note that NutriPath, a private Pathology lab in Victoria, presently carries out testing for the various lipoprotein subfractions.

LDL can now be separated into a maximum of seven LDL subfractions with what is called the "Liposcreen LDL-Subfractions Test". The LDL subfractions have been named LDL-1, consisting of the largest particles, through to LDL-7, consisting of the smallest particles.

Many individuals with normal LDL and HDL cholesterol levels remain at risk for coronary artery disease as the conventional tests do not convey the necessary detail. A Liposcreen profile quantifies the different subfractions.

See below for typical lipoprotein scans of a healthy PATTERN A lipoprotein pattern and an "at risk" PATTERN B individual:

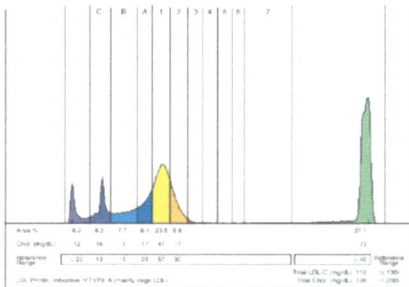

Figure 1. Typical *NORMAL* Liposcreen profile

Individuals exhibiting lipoprotein profiles, consisting primarily of the larger, buoyant LDL-1 and LDL-2 subfractions, have been designated as "Pattern A".

Pattern A is deemed a *NORMAL* lipoprotein pattern/profile.

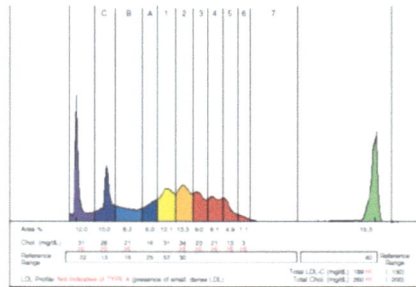

Figure 2. Typical *ABNORMAL* Liposcreen profile

Individuals exhibiting lipoprotein profiles, consisting primarily of the smaller and denser subfractions (LDL-3 through LDL-7) have been designated as "Pattern B"[5] .

Pattern B is deemed an *ABNORMAL* lipoprotein pattern/profile.

The PATTERN A (left hand) graph shows the normal lipoprotein fractions with the very low density (VLDL) and intermediate density peaks in purple and blue. The friendly low density (LDL) fractions 1 and 2 are shown in yellow and orange. The high density (HDL) lipoprotein fraction is seen in green.

The PATTERN B (right hand) graph shows an abnormal distribution with high levels of VLDL and IDL and the appearance of the dangerous LDL 3,4 5,6 and a trace of 7 which are shown in red and can be glycated/oxidized and promote coronary artery disease.

When a pathology lab looks at a person's LDL cholesterol it is often calculated, not measured. Lipoprotein fractionation allows you to understand which portion of the LDL particles are unhealthy, small dense LDL particles, prone to oxidation and glycation.

The following graph (Figure 1) from NutriPath shows that the dangerous LDL fractions 3 and 4 can be elevated even though the total cholesterol and triglycerides levels are well within the normal limits at 4.3 and 1.1 mmol/l respectively. Only fractionation of LDL would have spotted this.

Figure 1

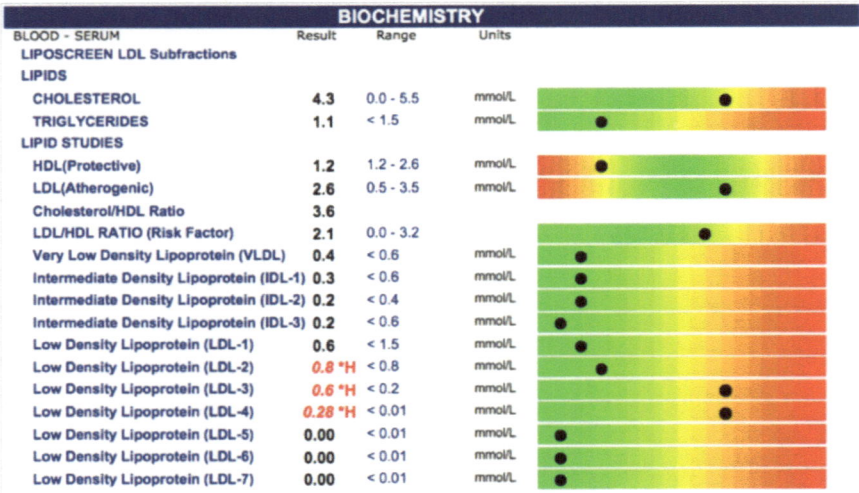

A total cholesterol of 6.3mmol/l (in Figures 2 and 3) is usually frowned upon by doctors and the patient would be prescribed a statin drug. However now we have more information. In the these following graphs we can see that the harmful LDLs 3,4,5,6 and 7 are all zero and thus the high cholesterol reading is not a risk factor because the LDLs reside in the harmless LDL 1 and 2 fractions.

Figure 2

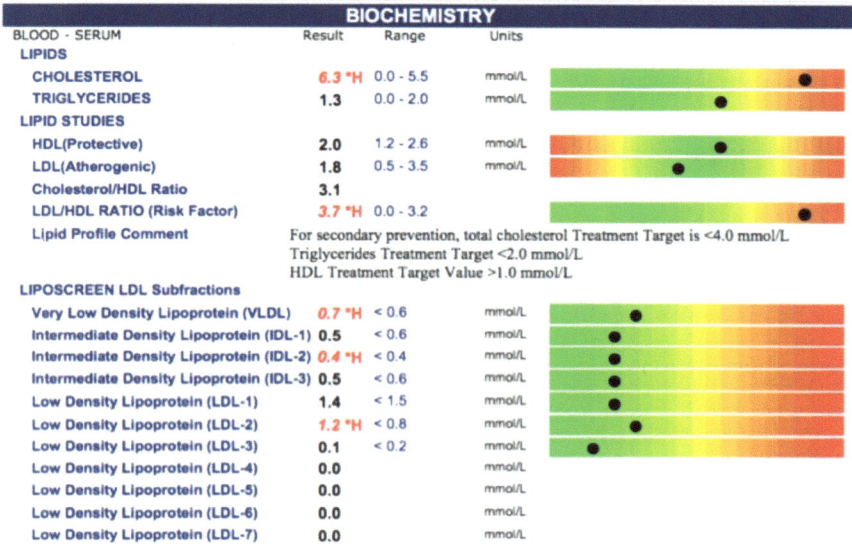

BIOCHEMISTRY				
BLOOD - SERUM	Result	Range	Units	
LIPIDS				
CHOLESTEROL	*6.3* *H	0.0 - 5.5	mmol/L	
TRIGLYCERIDES	**1.3**	0.0 - 2.0	mmol/L	
LIPID STUDIES				
HDL(Protective)	**2.0**	1.2 - 2.6	mmol/L	
LDL(Atherogenic)	**1.8**	0.5 - 3.5	mmol/L	
Cholesterol/HDL Ratio	**3.1**			
LDL/HDL RATIO (Risk Factor)	*3.7* *H	0.0 - 3.2		
Lipid Profile Comment	For secondary prevention, total cholesterol Treatment Target is <4.0 mmol/L			
	Triglycerides Treatment Target <2.0 mmol/L			
	HDL Treatment Target Value >1.0 mmol/L			
LIPOSCREEN LDL Subfractions				
Very Low Density Lipoprotein (VLDL)	*0.7* *H	< 0.6	mmol/L	
Intermediate Density Lipoprotein (IDL-1)	**0.5**	< 0.6	mmol/L	
Intermediate Density Lipoprotein (IDL-2)	*0.4* *H	< 0.4	mmol/L	
Intermediate Density Lipoprotein (IDL-3)	**0.5**	< 0.6	mmol/L	
Low Density Lipoprotein (LDL-1)	**1.4**	< 1.5	mmol/L	
Low Density Lipoprotein (LDL-2)	*1.2* *H	< 0.8	mmol/L	
Low Density Lipoprotein (LDL-3)	**0.1**	< 0.2	mmol/L	
Low Density Lipoprotein (LDL-4)	**0.0**		mmol/L	
Low Density Lipoprotein (LDL-5)	**0.0**		mmol/L	
Low Density Lipoprotein (LDL-6)	**0.0**		mmol/L	
Low Density Lipoprotein (LDL-7)	**0.0**		mmol/L	

Figure 3

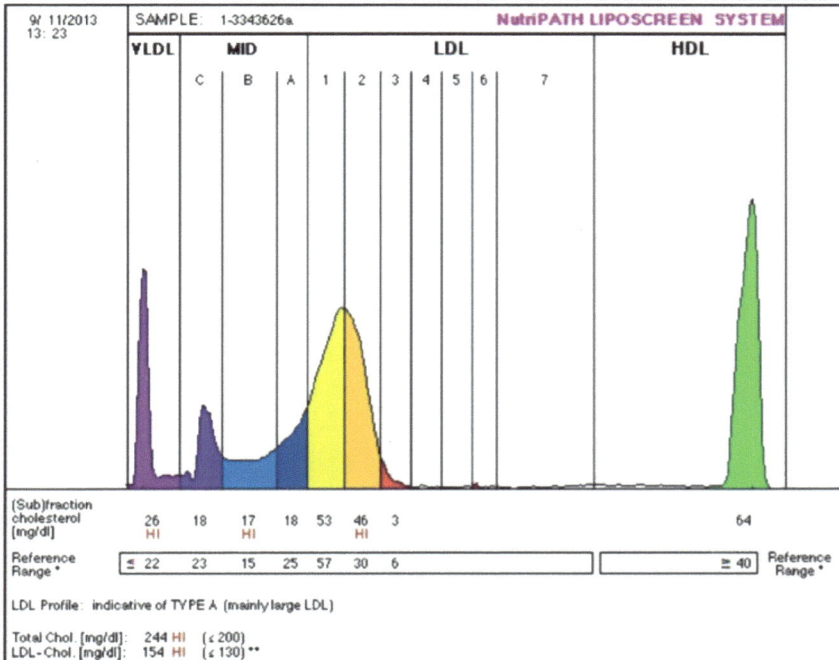

9/ 11/2013 13: 23   SAMPLE: 1-3343626a.   NutriPATH LIPOSCREEN SYSTEM

	VLDL	MID			LDL								HDL
		C	B	A	1	2	3	4	5	6	7		
(Sub)fraction cholesterol [mg/dl]	26 HI	18	17 HI	18	53 HI	46 HI	3						64
Reference Range *	≤ 22	23	15	25	57	30	6						≥ 40 Reference Range *

LDL Profile: indicative of TYPE A (mainly large LDL)

Total Chol. [mg/dl]: 244 HI   (< 200) **
LDL-Chol. [mg/dl]: 154 HI   (< 130) **

*Reference ranges derived from 125 serum samples that met the NCEP ATP III guidelines for desirable lipid status
**LDL-C is comprised of the sum of cholesterol in Mid bands C through A as well as all the subfractions

Other tests include Lipoprotein (a), Apolipoprotein B and Apolipoprotein A1. The ApoB level is rapidly becoming a more important indicator of coronary artery disease than cholesterol.

For more information on these and many other tests, NutriPath can be contacted at NutriPath PO Box 442, Ashburton VIC 3147 or email: info@nutripath.com.au or see website: http://www.nutripath.com.au.

There are now many laboratories worldwide which offer this type of specialized testing. These include:

- Quest Diagnostics have Diagnostic Laboratories worldwide http://www.questdiagnostics.com/home/about/locations.html
- http://www.questdiagnostics.com/testcenter/TestDetail.action?ntc=91604
- Atherotech http://thevaptest.com/
- Berkeley Heart Lab http://bhlinc.com/
- Lab Tests Online http://labtestsonline.org/understanding/analytes/lipoprotein-subfractions/tab/test/
- ImuPro Australia and New Zealand http://www.imupro.com.au/liposcan-test-practitioners
- Health Testing Centres http://www.healthtestingcenters.com/vap-cholesterol-test.aspx
- http://circ.ahajournals.org/content/119/17/2383.full
- http://www.drsinatra.com/cholesterol-tests/

Chapter 7: The Dietary Fat Connection

What type of fats do you consume? What do you buy at the supermarket, in bottles or hidden in processed foods? What fats and oils are in the meals you eat out? Most of us really can't answer these questions. So let's firstly have an in-depth look at the type of dietary fat that most people consume and examine more closely how this may affect the nature and composition of lipoproteins.

Key Points

- By largely removing stable animal fats, eggs, butter, cream and cheese from our diet and replacing them with unstable polyunsaturated oils, we have made a major change in the human diet.

- Essential fatty acid requirements of humans may be greatly overestimated.

- Saturated fat may not the bad guy it's made out to be.

- There's no food that's purely saturated fat. So called saturated fat is a mixture of fats.

- We eat far too much polyunsaturated oil.

- The ratio between polyunsaturated (PUFAs) and saturated fats has changed to become dangerous for human health.

- PUFAs are pro-inflammatory.

- PUFAs, in the form and quantities we ingest, are dangerous for our heart.

- Don't eat margarine!

As we discussed in the previous chapter, one of the most profound dietary changes of the last 50 years is the replacement of saturated fats with polyunsaturated fats. This change coincided with the scare campaign against saturated fat and spawned an industry of polyunsaturated oils now found in supermarkets including corn, soya, flaxseed, grape, sunflower and safflower oils. Not just small amounts, but litres of these oils now grace our kitchen shelves. We call them omega-6 oils because they contain a large percentage of omega-6 fatty acids.

Implications of Changing to Omega-6 PUFAs

By now you're familiar with the concept that a major problem with vegetable-derived dietary oils is that they are fragile and unstable. They are easily damaged by light, heat, air and deteriorate over time when packed in small clear glass or plastic containers. They are also heavily processed. The micronutrients that were initially associated with the oils in their natural state have been removed.

As previously mentioned, linoleic acid is the major ingredient in seed oils, present at over 50%-65% and around 75% in safflower oil. It's an "essential" omega-6 fatty acid, so-named because we cannot make it in the body. We need to include it in our diet. The question is how much and in what form?

Over tens of thousands of years our intake was sufficient by just eating animal and seafood fats with the addition of whole seeds, nuts and some vegetable-based fats. It's only during the last 50-60 years that we've been brainwashed into thinking that we must have huge quantities of oils every day. Our consumption patterns have blown out.

Keeping in mind the drastic effect that oxidation and inflammation can have on our arteries and the relationship with oxidized LDL and plaque formation, here are some other important things you should know about polyunsaturated oils:

- *The more polyunsaturated oils in a diet, the greater is the body's requirement for vitamin E and other fat soluble factors such as coenzyme Q10 to protect against the harmful effects of the oil.* Consuming large amounts of canola oil can cause a critical vitamin E deficiency.

- Problems with the oxidation of linoleic acid will be greater if there is a whole body deficit of important phytonutrients such as the carotenoids, flavonoids and other similar compounds normally present in a high fiber diet that is rich in fruit, vegetables, grains, sprouts and legumes. These small micronutrients are natural anti-inflammatory agents and antioxidants but are simply not present in many western diets composed largely of refined carbohydrates such as white flour and sugar products plus junk foods like french fries and soft drinks (sodas).

- Frying or baking with polyunsaturated oils can speed up the oxidation of linoleic acid. It oxidises quickly under heat to form linoleic acid hydroperoxide, one of the major toxins in atherosclerosis.

- Much research has now confirmed that linoleic acid *per se*, even before oxidation, may activate genes that produce inflammatory agents called chemokines and cytokines that cause injury to the blood vessel walls. This may be quite apart from its ability to form an unstable and oxidised molecule. (1)

- What about cold-pressed oils? Unfortunately, even the cold-pressed polyunsaturated seed oils will quickly oxidise at the ambient temperature inside the body.

- Oxidation happens more rapidly in the presence of blood or tissue-derived "free radicals" and in cases where iron and copper are not bound to plasma proteins in disorders like haemochromatosis or Wilson's disease.

- Scientific evidence indicates that linoleic acid is also a potent promoter of tumour growth. In the 1960s, interest in organ transplantation led to the discovery that polyunsaturated fats prolong graft survival by suppressing the immune system. The component that did this was more than likely linoleic acid. (2)

Trans Fats and Major Illness

You may be familiar with the term "trans fats". Through advertising, magazines, TV, the internet and general media many people are starting to get the idea that refined, hydrogenated seed oils can also contain dangerous substances called trans isomers/trans fatty acids or trans fats. These are formed when vegetable oils are "hydrogenated" or hardened to make margarine or shortening. Trans fats are now recognized as a leading cause of heart disease, cancer, diabetes, and other chronic or fatal illnesses. For this reason many manufacturers have started to produce products which are free of trans fats.

That's a change for the better *but don't think that by avoiding trans fats, you are avoiding all the toxic potential of polyunsaturated oils.*

And They're Still Selling Margarine

When I wrote my original book on the topic of cholesterol, nearly everyone was eating margarine instead of butter. Butter sales had slumped and margarine was doing very nicely. If you asked most people why they ate margarine they would say it was because they were "not allowed" to have butter as it contains saturated fat, while margarine contained the new wonder fats of the day, the polyunsaturates. What no one was talking about at the time was that margarine actually had the highest source of trans fatty acids.

Fortunately that picture is changing. People now understand that butter is a natural product. And the more natural you can find it, the better. That dark yellow surface that forms on a lump of butter that frequently goes in and out of the refrigerator is a sign of oxidation. Cut it off; don't eat it. Once again the advice seems to be to eat better quality and less. Butter is, after all, one of our few excellent sources of vitamin A.

So if you haven't caught up on the margarine debate yet, read a bit about its manufacture and make up your own mind. It's not just that margarine is made of polyunsaturated oils like sunflower, rapeseed, canola and soybean. It's what the manufacturing process does to the original product. Margarine is anything but natural. It would be difficult to find anything more processed. Firstly it's subject to extreme heat and pressure and usually extraction with solvents. It has to be squeaky "clean" so it's bleached. More heating and pressure and a few magic industrial additions turns the oily mess back into a semi-solid form (so spreadable!). The process used is called hydrogenation and it gives rise to those trans fats, which we now know are highly correlated with heart disease. Trans fats cause inflammation in the cells which line the arteries. Trans fats are so dangerous that manufacturers now have to list the content on packaging and fortunately many manufacturers are now eliminating them entirely.

These days margarine's promotional push has to do with the plant sterols which are added to help reduce cholesterol. A better way to get your sterols is to eat a small handful of fresh nuts or seeds most days.

Margarine manufacturers may also add omega-3s so the average customer is thinking they're getting the equivalent of taking fish oil capsules. However these additions are usually derived from cheaper vegetable sources, which are not particularly effective and can't really be compared with marine oils. The implication is mainly there to seduce the unwary buyer.

Those interested may like to read more research on the question of margarine and trans fats in the reference section:

- Butter verses margarine (3)
- 30,000 cardiac episodes per year in the US were attributed to the consumption of trans fats (4)

Omegas 3 and 6—The Ratio Makes the Difference

> Just for the record, a shorthand way of expressing omega-6 and
> omega-3 fatty acids is n-6 and n-3 fatty acids, respectively. It's a
> common abbreviation and useful for those without a scientific
> background who want to read the references and other source
> material.

Most people these days are aware of omega-3 oils. We know about the
importance of eating fatty fish and many of us are taking omega-3 fish oil
supplements on a daily basis. Not everyone understands why such interest
has grown over the last few decades. Are you aware, for example, that
humans have become very deficient in omega-3 oils relatively recently, as a
result of what is possibly the biggest uncontrolled unscientific study in
human history. We now live in a nutritional environment where fats and oils
differ dramatically from that in which our genetic constitution evolved. It's
unprecedented and hasn't happened in the last 2 million years of hunter
gatherer existence. We're only just learning about the side effects that have
come from our recent messing about with oils. We desperately need to get
back to balance, but for the time being we've lost it.

So what is a healthy balance between omega-3 and omega-6 oils? Well, it
used to be around 1:2. In early human history, omega-3 fatty acids were
found in all foods consumed including meat, fish, eggs, nuts, berries and wild
plants. Over the last 150 years the ratio of omega-3 to omega-6 essential fatty
acids in western diets has risen from 1:2 to about 1:20, largely due to the
increased consumption of polyunsaturated vegetable oils. That's right; the
ones in the supermarket.

The huge quantities of unstable supermarket oils, which we now consume,
are behind a massive increase in levels of omega-6 in the human diet.
Omega-6 oils have strong inflammatory effects. This move to omega-6 oils
has produced metabolites that contribute to the formation of blood clots,
atheroma (plaque), allergies and inflammatory disorders, depressed immune
function, sterility, cell proliferation, cancer and weight gain. These oils are
major contributors in the pathogenesis of many diseases including
cardiovascular disease, diabetes, arthritis, osteoporosis, cancer, mental
health, dry eye disease and age-related macular degeneration. Both omega-6
and omega-3 oils influence gene expression, so that changes we are making
to our diet now may be handed down for generations.

On the other hand omega-3 fatty acids have anti-inflammatory, anti-
thrombotic, anti-arrhythmic, hypolipidaemic, and vasodilatory properties.
A different set of metabolites is formed when the fat balance is changed back

to a normal ratio - less pain, clotting, allergies, inflammation and most of the above disorders.

The beneficial effects of omega-3 fatty acids have been shown in the secondary prevention of coronary heart disease, hypertension and type 2 diabetes. In the secondary prevention of cardiovascular disease, a ratio of 1:4 (omega-3:omega-6 oils) was associated with a 70% decrease in total mortality. Ideally public health policy should advise a move from our present ratio of 1:20 towards an ideal of 1:1 or 1:3. (5)

Omega-3, Cardiovascular Disease and Depression

Numerous studies have shown that omega-3 fatty acids reduce the risk of cardiac arrest or sudden cardiac death and that a high omega-6 to omega-3 ratio has been reported in the heart muscle of men following sudden cardiac death. Specifically, omega-3 fatty acids are thought to have anti-arrhythmic properties and an impact on heart rate variability.

In chapter 2 we talked about the importance of having cholesterol in cell membranes of the brain and CNS and how a reduction of cholesterol opens the flood gates for mood and other mental disorders. But could the well-known association between depression and cardiovascular disease be explained by a deficiency in omega-3 fatty acids?

In a recent study of patients with acute coronary syndrome, researchers found that those among them with major depression had significantly lower concentrations of omega-3 fatty acids such as DHA, as well as higher omega-6 to omega-3 ratios. This was thought to be the first study showing lower omega-3 levels in depressed patients with coronary artery disease, whereas numerous other studies had found low omega-3 levels in people who later developed coronary artery disease. (6)

Sources of Omega-3 Oils

Micro algae and other marine microorganisms are the natural omega-3 factories of the sea. They are prevalent in cold waters. If fish move from a cold sea environment to more tropical waters the omega-3 balance of their food supply changes and they incorporate more omega-6 oils into their bodies. The omega-3 balance will depend upon the food the fish are fed. Fish caught in tropical waters and fish that have no omega -3 food source will be deficient in omega-3 oils. This particularly applies to the farmed cold water fish which usually feed on a large percentage of dietary omega-3 oils but not if their usual source of food is cut off. The present popularity of krill oil, though an effective source of omega-3, may be unsustainable and detrimental to many species which rely on maintaining the ecosystems of the oceans.

Linseed (flaxseed) oil is also a good source of omega-3 oils but is not very well utilized by humans. Only a very small percentage (around 5-10%) is converted into the important EPA (eicosapentaenoic acid) and DHA (docosahexaenoic acid) which are vital for making many of the important substances which control all cell metabolism. These latter two important long chain polyunsaturated fatty acids are found in fish oils and are not found in land-based animals.

Monounsaturated Dietary Oils

Olive oil in its extra virgin state is a better choice of oil for everyday use. It has a higher balance of monounsaturated oil, is much more stable and contains many polyphenolic anti-inflammatory substances (which tend to prevent oxidation while in the bottle), including vitamin E. This is important because olive oil also contains 8-12% PUFAs and they need protecting.

Canola oil is also predominantly monounsaturated but like all modern vegetable oils, canola oil goes through the process of caustic refining, bleaching and degumming, all of which involve high temperatures or chemicals of questionable safety. Most of the high content of omega-3s in canola oil are transformed into trans fats during the deodorization process. (7)

Mixing It Together

Saturated fats may confer a protective effect on polyunsaturated fats. Interestingly, there is virtually no fat or oil-based food that does not contain a certain amount of both. Research continues to back this up. The saturated fats are highly protective. A better approach may be to combine moderate amounts of good quality vegetable oils with saturated fats. You will note that the Italians have been cooking with a mixture of butter and olive oil for years.

> ### Do you know why the seed oil market grew?
>
> Vegetable oils were initially used in paints and plastics. However other oil-based products replaced them after the Second World War. So, what to do with all this vegetable oil?
>
> Enter the Lipid Hypothesis of heart disease in the 50's—the fashionable idea was that high blood cholesterol caused atherosclerosis and polyunsaturated oils would lower blood cholesterol.
>
> So seed oils had found a new market—the prevention of heart disease!
>
> Pity that both animal and human studies were showing that these oils in large quantities were toxic to the heart and increased the incidence of cancer.

Story with an Unhappy Ending: The Prudent Diet

As a result of the presumed association between cholesterol and heart disease the American Heart Association (AHA) recommended the Prudent Diet in 1956, where corn oil, margarine, fish, chicken and cold cereal, replaced butter, lard, beef, potatoes and eggs.

While most members of the AMA were in favour of the Prudent Diet, one member, Dudley White, M.D. disagreed with his AHA colleagues. He pointed out from his experience that heart disease in the form of myocardial infarction (MI) was almost non-existent in 1900, when egg consumption was three times what it was in 1956 and when corn oil was unavailable.

> When pressed to support the Prudent Diet, AMA member Dudley White replied:
>
> "See here, I began my practice as a cardiologist in 1921, and I never saw a myocardial infarction (MI) patient until 1928. Back in the MI-free days before 1920, the fats were butter and lard, and I think we would all benefit from the kind of diet we had at a time when no one had ever heard the words "corn oil".

Nevertheless trials of the Prudent Diet went ahead. In 1957, Dr. Norman Jolliffe, director of the Nutrition Bureau of the New York Health Department, launched an Anti-Coronary Club for businessmen age 40 to 59.

All were placed on the Prudent Diet, and results were published in the *Journal of the American Medical Association* in 1966.

Those on the Prudent Diet did succeed in slightly lowering their cholesterol levels. They had an average serum cholesterol of 5.7mmol/l (220mg/dl), compared to 6.5mmol/l (250mg/dl) in the meat-and-potatoes control group. (8)

However, the study authors were obliged to note that *there were eight deaths from heart disease among Dr. Jolliffe's Prudent Diet group, and none among those who ate meat three times a day.* Dr. Jolliffe was dead by this time. He succumbed in 1961 from a vascular thrombosis, although the obituaries listed the cause of death as complications from diabetes.

Getting to Know Those Scary Saturated fats

Some key points:

- Saturated fatty acids (SFAs) are made in the body.
- Saturated fatty acids raise the friendly HDL.
- Saturated fatty acids lower atherogenic lipoprotein(a).
- Saturated fatty acids conserve useful omega-3 fatty acids.
- Saturated fatty acids do not inhibit insulin binding i.e. they're better for your blood sugar.

Animal fat composition tables show that

- what we commonly call saturated fat is mainly monounsaturated oleic acid,
- saturated palmitic and stearic acids and accounts for about 43% of total fat. The monounsaturated fat accounts for another 45-47%. (Yes, that's the same healthy monounsaturated fat that's in olive oil),
- the remainder is comprised of 3-10% PUFAs.

People had been taught to react with aversion to the words "saturated fat". If you started to ask some questions, you would find that saturated fatty acids (SFAs) are referred to as "saturated" because they are chemically stable. When it comes to oil, "stable" is a good thing. There are no chemical double bonds (which are very reactive and can oxidize very easily). Unlike PUFAs, there is very little possibility of rancidity or spoilage.

Saturated fats have been in the human diet for many thousands of years while heart disease at the turn of the last century was practically unheard of. Historically humans have predominantly eaten saturated fats and olive oil. PUFAs were available in smaller amounts in their pure form, particularly from nuts and seeds.

I remember a few years back when I was travelling in southern France we came upon fields of lambs grazing on the hilly flowering pastures outside a town called Sisteron. The fields were covered in spring herbs. When we ate the lamb over the next few days it was unbelievably delicious and tasted as if the lamb had been marinated in a strong herbal mixture. In reality natural pasture grazing had transferred herbal substances to the flesh of the lambs. Their fat was naturally "marinated" in antioxidants and other anti-inflammatory substances. As you will see, this is more than just an anecdotal holiday memory. The link between dietary sources of saturated fat and the total antioxidant availability both in the fat tissue and within the context of a whole meal is vital to the story as it unfolds.

A valuable part of this unfolding is the research promoted by Mary Enig and Sally Fallon, who, in conjunction with the Weston Price Foundation, have explored a long list of reasons why saturated fats are not artery clogging and do not cause heart disease. Possibly the reverse is true. They explain that "saturated 18-carbon stearic acid and 16-carbon palmitic acid are the preferred foods for the heart, which is why the fat around the heart muscle is highly saturated. The heart draws on this reserve of fat in times of stress." (9)

So is there any scientific evidence as to why we should be removing all the saturated fats from our diets? Where are the clinical trials and other studies showing a relationship between eating saturated fats and heart disease? In short there are none. There are, however, major studies showing that saturated fat does not cause heart disease.

The Experts' Decision on Saturated Fat Intake

The facts are that cardiovascular mortality has never been convincingly demonstrated to increase with saturated fat intake.

In 2009 the *Annals of Nutrition and Metabolism* dedicated a whole edition (Fats and Fatty Acids in Human Nutrition) to reporting an "Expert Consultation" held jointly by the World Health Organization (WHO) and Food and Agriculture Organization (FAO) of the US. The 2008 consultation took a wide, sweeping look at the relationship between fats, physiology and health. They started out with an assumed link between saturated fat and heart disease. You may be surprised about what they discovered. (10)

The "experts" responsible for assessing this relationship looked at two lines of evidence: epidemiological studies and intervention studies. Let's look at both in turn.

Epidemiological studies look at the relationship between factors such as smoking and lung cancer, exercise and dementia, SFAs and heart disease in populations. These studies can only really tell us about associations between things. They can't generally be used to inform us if one thing is causing another. Nevertheless, if saturated fat does truly cause heart disease (like we've been told for the last few decades), then the epidemiological evidence should show that higher levels of saturated fat are associated with a higher risk of heart disease (also known as "coronary heart disease" or "CHD" for short).

Not surprisingly the outcome of the report wasn't widely publicized. Essentially the WHO/FAO report could find little association. This is what they said:

> "Intake of SFA was not significantly associated with CHD mortality...
>
> and also:
>
> "SFA intake was not significantly associated with CHD events (e.g. heart attacks)..."

In *intervention studies* individuals are subjected to some sort of intervention (such as a medication, increased exercise or dietary change). The relevant intervention in this case was to put people on a low saturated fat diet, and see how they fared compared to individuals who were not subjected to this change. Unlike epidemiological studies, intervention studies can prove "causal" links between things. For example, if eating less saturated fat leads to a reduced risk of heart disease, then it's a pretty good bet that saturated fat causes heart disease (all other things being equal).

So, what did the WHO/FAO report find regarding relevant intervention studies? This is their conclusion:

> "...fatal CHD was not reduced by...the low-fat diets..."

Now let's look at another recent study which took the form of a meta-analysis. The material was published in March 2010 and assessed the relationship between saturated fat and heart disease. The study was an amalgamation of 21 epidemiological studies. Taken all together, this review monitored almost 347,747 people with 5 and 23 years of follow-up. (11)

And the findings?

- No association between saturated fat intake and risk of coronary heart disease.
- No association between saturated fat intake and risk of stroke.
- No association between saturated fat intake and cardiovascular disease.

> You know what all this means, don't you? That there is virtually no evidence that saturated fat causes heart disease or cardiovascular disease.

This was further substantiated during a symposium on saturated fats held in Copenhagen in May 2010. After the symposium the lead author of the proceedings and co-organizer Professor Arne Astrup said that replacing saturated fat with carbohydrates does not reduce the risk of coronary heart disease and may even further increase the risk. (12)

The justification for the anti-saturated fat campaign that has raged on for half a century is largely baseless.

Even if saturated fat were to increase LDL, it increases protective HDL right along with it.

Lastly, two Boston researchers examined all the scientific literature for a possible role of saturated fat in the incidence of heart disease, stroke and diabetes. *They found that the health effects of reducing saturated fat depended upon what nutrients replaced the fat.*

Like Professor Astrup, they found that if the saturated fat was replaced with the most common nutrient, which is carbohydrate, there was no benefit.

Replacing saturated fat with monounsaturated fat produced "uncertain effects" and although recommendations to replace saturated fats with polyunsaturated fats might appear appropriate, the much larger cardiovascular disease burdens caused by other dietary factors (e.g., low omega-3, low fruits and vegetables, high trans fat, and high salt) appeared to warrant much more attention. (13)

> **Did You Know?**
>
> "The more saturated fat you eat, the less likely you are to suffer an (ischaemic) stroke.
>
> Your risk of stroke decreases by 15% for every 3% increase in your saturated fat intake".

The Composition of Saturated Fats

Until recently it has been assumed that all saturated fats are associated with cardiovascular disease and therefore bad for you. Likewise it was assumed that the consumption of foods containing saturated fat would cause an increase in LDL cholesterol.

When we talk about saturated fat you may get the impression that there is only one type of fat present. This is not so. (14) In fact, the saturated fat from our main food sources such as beef, lamb, eggs, pork and butter is predominantly composed of oleic acid. It's around 45% oleic acid-the same healthy stuff found in olive oil. It's good for you. Other components are palmitic acid and stearic acid with a small percentage of myristic acid and lauric acid. Each of these different monounsaturated and saturated fats has a different effect on the lipoprotein fractions in our blood.

The negative assumptions around saturated fat remain largely unproven. For example, in 2003 researchers, Mensink and colleagues, combined the results of 60 carefully controlled dietary studies into a meta-analysis to confirm that LDL cholesterol and total cholesterol were not increased by consumption of stearic acid. However, neither did it increase HDL cholesterol. So here was a direct confirmation of a wide range of studies showing that stearic acid was basically innocuous in that it had no effect at all on lipoprotein levels. (15)

This study also revealed that the other saturated fat components-palmitic, myristic and lauric acids-did in fact increase LDL cholesterol, but at the same time they increased HDL cholesterol. So the HDL-raising effect is significant and more than compensates for the rise in LDL.

With the growing realization that high levels of functional HDL are protective against heart disease, this is an interesting finding.

This study was repeated by the USDA Beltsville (Maryland) Human Nutrition Research Centre, where they compared stearic acid against other dietary fats and confirmed the results.

This research should make most people pause and consider. If we look at animal fat composition tables we see no scientific evidence linking saturated fatty acids with heart disease risk-with the possible exception of palmitic acid. As we just mentioned, even though palmitic acid raises LDL, it also raises the HDL, which is protective against heart disease.

Balancing Saturated and Polyunsaturated Fats

Current thinking suggests that understanding the balance between the polyunsaturated fatty acid, linoleic acid, and saturated fat may start to give us some real answers about what is a cardio friendly fat profile. The presence of small amounts of linoleic acid (4.5%) in the diet actually gives even more protection against cholesterol elevation.

When it comes to palmitic acid, it's interesting to consider that maintaining a sufficient level of essential PUFAs may balance out even any slight negative effect of this saturated fatty acid on cholesterol elevation. French and colleagues did a study on this. Healthy individuals were fed palmitic acid as 10% of their daily energy needs while at the same time decreasing the polyunsaturated oil content by removing linoleic acid.

Results showed that as the linoleic acid level was removed from the diet, cholesterol synthesis increased. High levels of palmitic acid did not increase cholesterol production as long as the linoleic acid in the diet was greater than 4.5% energy. The linoleic acid/palmitic acid balance controlled the cholesterol production. When the diet replaced palmitic acid with trans fatty acids however, total cholesterol and LDL cholesterol increased with a decrease in HDL cholesterol. (16)

This concept of having a balance between the saturated fat intake and polyunsaturated fat intake is further reinforced by a recent study involving 59 men and women who were given emulsified drinks of palm stearin (the solid component of palm oil containing palmitic acid 59%, stearic acid 5%, oleic 28% and linoleic acid 6%) with and without a similar quantity of omega-3 oil added (which was predominantly the polyunsaturated long chain fatty acid, DHA).

The addition of the omega-3 oils to the drink completely reversed a reduction in blood flow bought on by the pure palm stearin. Palm stearin is a much more concentrated form of saturated fat than either beef fat or lard.

Note from the table below that it has 59% palmitic acid ,which is more than double the amount in beef fat or lard. The neutral stearic acid content is only 5%. This is less than half the amount in animal fats. Also the heart friendly oleic acid is less in the palm oil than beef fat.

It should be noted that while palmitic acid may decrease blood flow in the short term, it was separated from the usual balance of stearic, oleic and linoleic and because of its HDL elevating effect, may not be expected to be a risk factor for heart disease in the long term. (17)

You can see from these numbers that when you increase the intake of saturated palmitic acid in the diet while decreasing the friendly or neutral stearic and oleic acids, blood flow is negatively affected.

With an appropriate balance of linoleic acid (greater than 4.5% energy) or adding omega-3 oils at a ratio of 1:1, the so-called harmful saturated fats suddenly become CARDIO-FRIENDLY.

"Greater than 4.5%" linoleic acid is not the same as 30% of the total energy content of the diet. This is why it is so important not to use huge quantities of the polyunsaturated seed oils on a daily basis. Better a handful of nuts or avocado in your salad.

Obviously we need small quantities but these should be balanced with some saturated fats from animals and also omega-3 oils.

Some Positive Dietary Advice

Add some healthy sources of linoleic acid to your meals by eating a few nuts or seeds with animal protein. You could try a pesto sauce (pinenuts, walnuts) or some slivered almonds tossed with a stir fry.

The composition of the fatty acids in animal fat and palm oil is typically as follows:

	Beef Fat	Lard	Palm Oil
Saturated fatty acids:			
Palmitic acid	26%	25-28%	59%
Stearic acid	14%	12-14%	5%
Myristic acid	3%	1%	1%
Monounsaturated fatty acids:			
Oleic acid	47%	44-47%	28%
Palmitoleic acid	3%	3%	
Polyunsaturated fatty acids:			
Linoleic acid	3%	6-10%	6%
Linolenic acid	1%		

Note: Omega-3 oils found in grass fed meat include alpha linolenic acid, EPA, DHA, DPA and can comprise 2-5% of total beef fatty acids.

Why Pasture Fed Beef is Superior to Grain Fed Beef

While we are talking about the fatty acid balance in the diet we should compare the balance in grain fed verses grass fed beef. Many people are not aware that there is a huge difference in the fatty acid and nutrient composition between the two.

Feedlots are designed to maximize weight and minimize costs. Grass fed animals are definitely the healthiest for human nutrition. It's not just the superior feed, but also the extra exercise and lower stress levels that impact on the quality of the meat, which is directly linked to human cholesterol profiles.

> Pasture fed beef has a lower fat content than the grain fed beef as well as a higher proportion of stearic acid which has a neutral effect on lipoprotein levels.

The leaner pasture fed beef also tends to reduce LDL concentrations in both normal individuals and those with higher levels of cholesterol.

Animal studies have also shown that grass fed beef produce fat with more conjugated linoleic acid. This is formed by bacteria in the stomachs of herbivores such as cows.

Cows allowed to graze freely in pastures, and not fed with supplements of corn silage or corn oil, had 500% more conjugated linoleic acid in their milk fat than cows fed typical dairy diets. (18)

Conjugated linoleic acid is a natural polyunsaturated fatty acid compound found in many foods, including milk, cheese, and meats. The meat that is richest in conjugated linoleic acid is beef. Research is presently under way into its many anticipated health benefits including in the areas of cancer, atherosclerosis, obesity and diabetes.

Conjugated linoleic acid has been shown (in hamsters) to:

- reduce levels of LDL
- reduce levels of triglycerides
- improve the ratio of LDL to HDL
- improve the ratio of total cholesterol to HDL
- conserve vitamin E, a major antioxidant in fat metabolism, as indicated by a higher vitamin E to cholesterol ratio. (19)

Grass fed beef has much higher levels of monounsaturated fatty acids and PUFAs. The intramuscular marbling is less than in grain fed beef but this is compensated for by the higher level of monounsaturated fat.

Omega-3 fatty acid levels are also consistently higher in grass fed beef compared to their grain fed counterparts. Omega-3 oils found in grass fed meat include alpha-linolenic acid, EPA, DHA, DPA and can comprise 2-5% of total beef fatty acids. It may vary depending on the type of pastures the beef are grazing on. (20)

If we are trying to improve the ratio of omega 3 to omega 6 oils in our diet, grass fed beef is the better choice of meat.

Humans benefit directly from the quality of meat they consume. Beef consumption can significantly increase serum concentrations of a number of omega-3 fatty acids including, EPA, DPA and DHA.

Did You Know?

Almost everyone in the 21st century suffers from an imbalance of omega 3 and omega 6 fatty acids.

Omega-3 and omega-6 fatty acids are two separate families of fats but they share the same enzymes during their metabolism.

An imbalance in the ratio can interfere with the final end-products and this can have serious ramifications for health.

Enzymes favour omega-3 fatty acids before the omega-6. This may indicate how important the omega-3s are.

The Taste Test

In comparison studies grass fed beef was found to taste better, probably because of the animals' diverse diet.

Vitamin/Antioxidant Levels in Grass-fed Beef

Cattle that are pasture fed pick up different phytonutrients from grasses, shrubs, clover, hay, silage and wild herbs. They have carcass fat that is more yellow than their grain fed counterparts. This diverse diet is also behind the superior taste associated with grass fed animals. This is caused by the carotenoids from the green forages. Concentrations were 0.45 µg/g and 0.06 µg/g for beef from pasture and grain fed cattle respectively. That's a 7 fold increase in beta-carotene levels for grass fed beef over their grain fed cousins.

Beta carotene is converted into vitamin A in the body. Vitamin A deficiency in humans is a growing concern.

Grass fed beef is also richer in nutrients including vitamin E, K and B complex, flavonoids, magnesium, calcium, potassium and trace elements.

Vitamin E levels are also significantly higher in pasture fed animals and range from 0.75 to 2.92 micrograms/gram of muscle in the grain fed verses 2.1 to 7.73 micrograms/gram in the pasture fed beef depending on the type of forage. This increased vitamin E level in pasture fed beef extends shelf life by delaying oxidative deterioration which gives a brown appearance to the meat.

Glutathione levels are particularly high in grass fed animals. This is one of the most important antioxidants in the body. It is made up of 3 amino acids including cysteine, glutamic acid and glycine. It knocks out free radicals like hydrogen peroxide and protects cells from oxidized lipids and proteins and prevents damage to DNA.

Other key antioxidant enzymes such as superoxide dismutase (SOD) and catalase are also higher in pasture-fed beef. SOD and catalase are coupled enzymes that work together as powerful antioxidants. SOD scavenges superoxide anions by forming hydrogen peroxide and catalase then decomposes the hydrogen peroxide to water and oxygen.

Even though you may still mostly choose lean cuts of beef where the cutaneous fat has been trimmed, don't necessarily always shy away from the tasty intramuscular marbling from meat which has been grass fed.

> Grass-only diets improve the oxidative enzyme concentration in beef, protecting the muscle lipids against oxidation as well as providing the beef consumer with an additional source of antioxidant compounds.

Old-fashioned Cows

Dairy products were only introduced during the last 7,000 years and this may explain why so many people are sensitive to some of the protein components and lactose, the milk sugar. However, many problems with dairy product metabolism may be the direct result of the way we process these products. Many communities ferment milk into yoghurt or other fermented products which are digested more easily and do not create a problem.

Cheese production has a long history and is an example of how fermentation has made many of the milk proteins accessible to our digestive processes where the milk starting material has proven to be a problem.

Many people nowadays can eat cheese and yoghurt but not drink milk.

In supermarkets there is now a strain of milk (called A2 milk in Australia) that is made from a species of cow that dates back to the pre-domestication of cattle. This milk comes from the strain *bos indicus* (which include humped cattle and buffalo) and not the usual *bos taurus* (which are the breed of most domesticated cows).

A2 milk has high levels of beta-casein A2 which have been shown to cause fewer problems in the causation of heart disease and diabetes because it does not contain a peptide called beta casomorphin-7 which has been implicated in these two disorders.

"Populations that consume milk containing high levels of beta- casein A2 variant, have a lower incidence of cardiovascular disease and Type-1 Diabetes. Furthermore consumption of milk with the A2 variant may be associated with less severe symptoms of autism and schizophrenia." (21)

Beta-casein A1 from the milk of the domesticated *bos taurus* variety of cow is far less friendly and has been associated with hardening of the arteries. According to Tailford and colleagues "...beta-casein A2 has a mildly atheroprotective effect while beta-casein A1 is most definitely atherogenic (causes hardening of the arteries). These results are consistent with epidemiological studies that suggest a strong relationship between mortality from cardiovascular disease and consumption of beta-casein A1, even though other studies show no association between reported milk consumption *per se* and cardiovascular mortality".(22)

So choosing the correct type of milk from a non-domesticated breed of cow and also adding friendly bacteria, can make a huge difference to the digestibility of milk products that we can consume today. It is not within the scope of this book to discuss the advantages and disadvantages of raw milk, but the reader may like to follow up on this discussion elsewhere.

Feeding the Chicken to Get the Best Egg

We have read a lot in the media lately about the way animals we eat are housed and fed. We have stories of chickens that are supposed to be "free range" living in confined conditions where two chickens are only given one square metre of land. This is not free range. We also have tragic stories of battery chickens, fed antibiotics, hormones and having bones that break so easily that the dead birds need to be cleared each morning. It could be different and indeed, change is starting to come about as consumers educate themselves and start to vote with their shopping choices.

Take this piece of research for example. Israeli researchers from the Institute for Nutrition Research, Rabin Centre, at Beilinson Hospital in Petach-Tikva, Israel, recently showed that the fatty acid composition in the eggs depended upon the grain composition of the feed given to the chickens. By designing wheat, barley and milo-based chicken feeds and replacing the soy/corn oils with canola they were able to increase the amount of antioxidants in the eggs produced and also reduce the unstable, inflammation causing omega-6 oil content.

What the team came up with is another example of a new industry of "designer" or "functional foods", the type we may look forward to in the future. They were able to reduce the omega-6 content of the egg from 22% to 12-15% and this resulted in a reduction in LDL oxidation of 36%.

In commenting on this result the researchers said, "We know that the combination of polyunsaturated fatty acids, especially (omega-6) like linoleic acid, is very prone to oxidation and LDL oxidation is a risk factor for atherosclerosis."

This research into eggs is set to expand. The leader of the Israeli research group, Dr Niva Shapira, noted that her future projects will be aimed at designing a nutrient profile for specific disease risks and developmental periods such as perinatal, preconception, during pregnancy and lactation and up to the ages 2-4 years old. "Eggs are among the best value for money protein and basic food, more sustainable and friendly with the environment, and easier to adapt to climate change and to acquire the knowledge of production in new populations."

Did You Know?

"Research shows that there is absolutely no connection between eating eggs and the risk of heart disease or stroke in either men or women." (23)

How Many Eggs Should I Eat?

If you're a middle-aged or elderly egg eater, don't skip this section.

Researchers from the University of Connecticut reported on a study of people in your age group in early April at the Experimental Biology meeting in San Francisco in 2006. (24)

Egg eating improved the quality of the cholesterol these people manufactured. Good quality cholesterol is what we're after. When people ate three or more eggs per day their bodies made bigger LDL- and HDL-lipoprotein particles than when they ate no eggs. That's important. As we've already pointed out, larger LDLs are less dangerous and less likely than smaller ones to enter artery walls and contribute to artery-clogging plaque. Similarly, larger HDLs are more robust than smaller ones at hauling cholesterol out of the blood vessel walls and, ultimately, out of the body.

Probably in response to this news release, in June 2006 an Australian TV personality, Dr Andrew Rochford, put his medical know-how where his mouth is when he decided to see what would happen to his blood cholesterol level when he ate 4 eggs each day for two weeks. Andrew's starting total cholesterol level was a low 3.8 mmol/l. The Australian Heart Foundation now like people to have cholesterols under 4.0 mmol/l.

After 2 weeks of eating 4 eggs per day, his cholesterol actually fell under 3.8mmol/l to such an extent that the monitor had no reading for it. At the same time an 18 year old body builder called Oscar McGill who was training for the world championships and eating 18 eggs per day also had his cholesterol level taken. Rather than his cholesterol reading being way off the scale, he also showed a low cholesterol reading.

So much for assuming that eggs increase cholesterol. Here is a perfect example of how a high cholesterol diet based on eating eggs actually turns off your own manufacture of cholesterol and this leads to a lower blood cholesterol level. So one of the best ways to lower your cholesterol while increasing the size of the LDL and HDL fractions (which are cardioprotective) is to eat eggs. But once again, it pays to go for quality and the most naturally produced foods available. *It also pays to go for moderation so most people won't want to imitate the above examples.*

A Final Word: A Big Tick for Saturated Fats

While I was submitting this book for publication one of the biggest reviews and meta-analysis published to date has put a final dampener on the push for more polyunsaturated fatty acids in our diet and gives saturated fats a well deserved breather.

This study by Dr Rajiv Chowdhury pooled the results of 72 studies that included 32 observational studies with 530,525 participants looking at dietary fatty acid intake; 17 observational studies of fatty acid biomarkers with 25,721 participants and 27 randomized controlled trials (103,052 participants) of fatty acid supplementation.

These researchers found no evidence that saturated fat increases the risk of coronary heart disease. Nor did they find that polyunsaturated fats have a cardioprotective effect. This detailed and extensive piece of research will most certainly prompt further study. (25)

Chapter 8: Sugar is the Hidden Enemy

Key Points

- Sugar causes more problems with cholesterol and heart disease than fat.

- Sugar is converted to fat (including cholesterol) inside the body.

- Limit your fructose intake to 2-3 pieces of whole fruit per day.

- Avoid high fructose corn syrup (HFCS) in all its form. Read labels carefully.

- Fructose intake is highly correlated with kidney disease.

- Avoid cooking at high temperatures.

- Common table sugar is made up of 50% fructose and 50% glucose.

Most people know that sugar isn't particularly good for their waistline. Fewer know it's bad for their health. One of the big dietary changes of the 20th century has been the separation of sugar from its original food source. Sugar now comes in different processed forms, not all equal. Enter the fructose story.

Around 500 years ago there were very few sources of fructose in the diet and such foods represented a minor component of daily intake. Examples would have included honey, dates, raisins, molasses, figs and fresh fruits in season such as grapes, apples and berries. Blueberries, for example, contain only 5-10% fructose by weight. These foods were still in their whole form with their micronutrients and fibre intact. They had not been cultivated for sweetness like today's blueberries, and were in fact more bitter and sour in their original form. These days we are all too inclined to separate fructose from the original food, then refine and concentrate it for mass production in the food industry.

Dietary patterns over the last 40-50 years have also been particularly marked by the steadily increasing consumption of sugar, both in the form of sucrose (common table sugar) and fructose (also known as fruit sugar). Fructose is sweeter than sucrose and this is one of the reasons it's now used so extensively as a sweetening agent in refined and processed foods, even in those labeled as health foods and organic.

So what's the problem with fructose? After all, it doesn't stimulate insulin release like glucose. The problem is that it heads straight to the liver where it is converted into fat. Interesting, when you consider that fructose and high fructose corn syrup (HFCS)-laden powders and beverages are used extensively in the weight loss industry. Could these products actually be facilitating weight gain rather than weight loss? Many of the low fat foods presently offered in the supermarkets are also loaded with fructose to replace the fat. No wonder it's so hard to lose weight by dieting with meal replacements containing fructose, sucrose or HFCS.

Drinking Your "Fructose Hit"

If you listen to good dietary advice you will hear that you need to be aware of the number of calories you get from what you drink. Fruit juices, soft drinks (sodas), sweetened tea and coffee, alcohol, etc. together with sucrose, fructose and high fructose corn syrup (HFCS) are difficult to avoid unless your main drink is water. Fifty percent of preschool children now consume some calorie-sweetened beverage every day. Some never drink water. *This "fructose hit"—the daily consumption of sweetened drinks—is a major change in the carbohydrate consumption of millions of people.*

It's not just about the calories. Could this change in sugar consumption patterns be fuelling both the obesity epidemic and the comorbidities linked to heart disease? So it would seem. Do we need to take this seriously? When conservative institutions like The American Heart Association start recommending that only 5% of daily calories should be consumed as added sugar (which is way down on the Dietary Guidelines for Americans 2010), it would have to get you thinking.

See the next chapter for some healthier beverage options.

Silent Killer?

Those in the know are aware that sugar is a silent killer. Sucrose and fructose are being widely exposed as key players in the development of heart disease, hypertension, obesity, diabetes, metabolic syndrome and even kidney disease. Consumption of fructose and sucrose at today's high levels appears to be a major cause of our current epidemic of heart disease—high triglycerides, high uric acid, high blood pressure, impaired glucose tolerance and insulin resistance. High blood levels of uric acid are an independent predictor of hypertension in 15 out of 16 studies and also of obesity and renal dysfunction. The high incidence of obesity, hypertension, diabetes, kidney and heart disease in African Americans is thought to be due to their higher intake of sugar and fructose and subsequently higher blood levels of uric acid.

Here are a few research studies that might alert you to what researchers from behind the scenes are finding. They show how sugar is converted to fat in the body and that sugar causes damage to that fat, and this is one of the greatest risk factors for heart disease.

Animal studies: When baboons were fed either high starch, fructose, glucose or sucrose all groups showed an increase in serum triglycerides ranging from 37% in the starch fed group to 65% in the fructose fed group. Cholesterol was increased in all groups and there was a reduced conversion of cholesterol into bile acids and increased fat stores in the liver. *All animals developed fatty plaque in their arteries but it was greatest in the fructose fed group.* (1)

Hampsters fed a high fructose diet developed fatty livers, hyperinsulinaemia and hyperlipoproteinaemia. (2)

Massachusetts Institute of Technology: Human studies demonstrated that high fructose consumption lead to increased blood fats, increased fat deposition in tissues and insulin resistance. Triglycerides increased over 75% after short term fructose feeding. The sensitivity of insulin decreased by 27%. (3)

A Swiss study in 2007 found that overweight children 6-14 years of age who consumed seriously high levels of fructose from sweets and sweetened drinks had much higher blood levels of triglycerides, lower HDL-cholesterol and increased numbers of smaller size LDL particles. It's critical information because these are the smaller LDL particles that represent one of the major risk factors for heart disease and high levels are directly related to the total fructose intake. These children are being primed for a future heart attack by consuming large quantities of fructose. (4)

Triglycerides: Did you Know?

The 25% of the population with the highest triglyceride to HDL ratio has 16 times more chance of a heart-related event than the 25% whose ratios were lowest. High triglycerides come from excess refined starches and sugar in the diet. (5)

Likewise, another recent study of 48 young overweight and normal weight adults found that participants consuming 25% of energy as glucose or fructose-sweetened beverages had some profound changes in their fat metabolism. The fructose group showed increased fat production in the liver, increased production of the dangerous small LDL, oxidized LDL and a short term increase in the synthesis of small triglyceride and cholesterol packages in the blood stream. In addition, blood glucose and insulin levels increased and insulin sensitivity decreased in subjects consuming fructose but not glucose. So glucose came out as less problematic than fructose in this study. (6)

Kidney Disease and Uric Acid—The Sugar Connection

Today there are 20 million Americans with stage 1 kidney disease and sugar (particularly fructose) is coming up as the number one cause of this growing epidemic. The mechanism appears to also involve an increase in uric acid. We usually think of uric acid in connection with gout but it is now thought to play a major role in hypertension, obesity, metabolic syndrome and the subsequent development of kidney disease.

Uric acid reduces nitric oxide in the blood vessel walls. Nitric oxide usually causes dilation of blood vessels. Uric acid causes constriction instead and leads to elevation of blood pressure. Uric acid also increases insulin, insulin resistance and triglyceride secretion by the liver. (7)

The Problem of Advanced Glycation End Products (AGEs)

It's normal for sugars to attach to fats and proteins in our body. It's a part of our normal metabolism. This type of attachment is usually controlled by an enzyme in a process called glycosylation and has a specific purpose.

Glycation is something different. This process is also about the bonding of a sugar molecule such as fructose or glucose to a protein or fat. However, glycation doesn't require an enzyme and is a random event that destroys the original function of the molecule. A new entity, or "glycated product" is created and is often implicated in heart disease and other age-related chronic diseases.

Glycated products are often referred to as advanced glycation end products (AGEs) and they play a critical role in ageing, atherosclerosis and long term vessel disorders in diabetes because of their connection to small LDL particles.

Figure 4: Formation of Advanced Glycation End Products

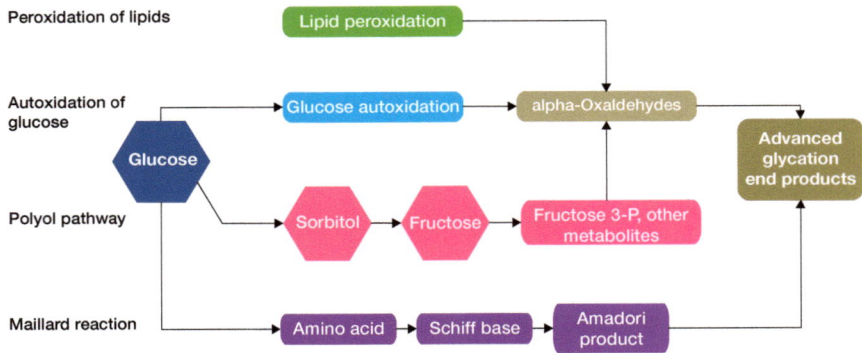

These advanced glycated products can also react with collagen in the blood vessel walls. This can cause stiffening of the blood vessels, high blood pressure or even micro- or macro-aneurisms that can lead to stroke. Glycated products can also react with fibrinogen to interfere with clotting.

Diabetics understand their haemoglobin glycated (HbA1c) due to the chronic presence of high blood sugar, and the degree of glycation, is often used as a measure of chronic sugar load in the blood.

Dangers of High Temperature Cooking

Just removing sugars from your diet will not necessarily prevent your body from accumulating glycated products. You also have to consider the way you cook. This is because glycated products and AGEs form when food high in protein and fat is cooked at high temperatures, especially in the presence of sugar. This applies to food that is barbecued, grilled or fried. Even oven roasted foods will be high in glycated products, especially if sugar is added.

Chefs often add sugar to the outside of a cake and other baked goods to get the browning reaction. This is also called the Maillard reaction named after a French chemist and is due to a heat-induced chemical reaction between amino acids in the protein and sugar. Of course it makes the foods taste delicious. It's found on top of your crème brulee or on glazed meat such as roast duck. It can be induced by basting with any of the popular marinades, as they usually contain sugar. You'll also see it in fried onions, roasted coffee and malted barley. French fries, potato chips, toasted bread, biscuits and brioche all contain AGEs. In 2002 scientists in Sweden accidentally discovered a very dangerous substance called acrylamide in starchy foods that had been heated. It was not found in food that had been boiled or in foods that were not heated.

If you want to cut down on ingesting AGEs or glycated products you need to stop cooking foods using intense heat. Don't bake under high, dry heat. Slower, cooler cooking techniques can get around the problem. Try poaching, steaming, braising, stewing and slow cooking, such as in a crockpot. Cook with fluids such as a broth or wine. Techniques like steaming and poaching prevent the formation of glycotoxins and other potential gene-mutating agents such as acrylamide.

Asian steam fry cooking involves sauteing food briefly in a wok with a little oil and then adding water, stock or wine and covering the pot. This stops the temperature rising above boiling point of water at 100 degrees centigrade. While there is water in the mix the temperature is kept below 100 degrees. This will minimize the formation of unwanted by-products.

Some Positive Dietary Advice

These findings indicate that we should drastically cut down on added sugar in our diet. Read all packets carefully to make sure they do not contain fructose, HFCS or sucrose. Be similarly alert to the presence of honey, agave, maltitol, etc. Take care eating out as many restaurants add hidden sugar to their dishes, particularly sauces and dressings. Eliminate highly refined, high GI flour, cakes, biscuits, breads, breakfast cereals, muffins, bagels, pasta, crackers and chips.

When we talk about harmful carbs we are really talking about processed sugars and starches. We are not talking about whole seasonal vegetables (which contains no fructose), legumes or whole fruit. The best fruits are those with low GI and which are highly coloured such as red, blue or purple coloured berries including blueberries, blackberries, raspberries, mulberries, strawberries, cherries, cranberries, black currants, acai, maqui and dark grapes. These are loaded with the very antioxidants and anti-inflammatory substances which will protect your cholesterol-carrying lipoproteins from oxidation.

How Much Sugar Do You Consume?

In 1995 about 68kg /year of HFCS was used in foods and beverages. This statistic has risen steadily ever since.

Fifteen years ago the average daily added sugar consumption was around 80g/day. Half of this was fructose. More importantly, the top 10% of consumers at this time, consumed 178g/day sucrose. Intake has increased consistently since then.

Chapter 9: Superfoods for Heart Disease and Cholesterol Management

The scientific research of the 20th century confirmed the use of many traditional practices in the field of health care. Such research indicated that we should reconsider the value of many foods known since antiquity, rather than have our total focus on new hi-tech products, many of dubious nutritional merit.

Our genes have changed very little in the last hundreds of thousands of years, so it stands to reason that what our ancestors ate may in fact be the best way to nourish ourselves. This is why we continue to see growing interest in the Mediterranean and paleolithic diets. Many are returning to traditional preparation practices such as stockmaking and food fermentation. Organically grown foods and farmers' markets have never been so popular as people en masse take greater interest in the quality of the food their families consume.

> Cereal grains products, dairy products, sweet beverages, seed oils, pre-packaged dressings, sugar and confectionary now comprise 60-70% of the energy in Western diets. The hunter-gatherer was exposed to virtually none of these foods.

Within the field of natural medicine the consumption of whole unprocessed foods has always been recommended but we now have the research support to streamline these choices in order to reduce a particular health problem and enhance some desired metabolic change. If, for example, olive oil lowers LDL-cholesterol and raises HDL-cholesterol while monounsaturated margarine containing trans-isomers does just the reverse, surely olive oil is the right food to choose. Garlic lowers blood lipids, protects vessel walls from harmful free radicals and tends to help dissolve clots due to its fibrinolytic action (chilli peppers have the same action). Ginger helps control platelet stickiness and hence thrombosis. The Thai people, for example, have very little thrombosis, mainly because of this beneficial action of such foods. I often advise my patients to increase the use of garlic, onions and hot peppers and ginger in cooking. The Japanese eat natto, which has fibrinolytic action and the choice of many as an alternative to drugs.

Evidence that communities that eat plenty of seafood have a lower incidence of cardiovascular disease is well-established. The question in the twenty first century is not whether we should eat seafood regularly, but how to do that in ways that are sustainable, affordable and natural. Mercury is becoming a big problem and many farmed fish do not have the same levels of omega-3 fatty acids in their tissue as their open-water cousins.

Whole grains have been in our diet for about ten thousand years. Except for people with gluten sensitivity, they are now known to be one of the best sources of natural fibres, trace elements and slow release glucose—all factors which have a protective function against the development of cardiovascular disease. Refined flours, sugars and foods containing them, on the other hand, do not have fibre, do not contain phytonutrients, vitamins and trace elements and do not induce the same stabilisation of blood sugars.

Cooked whole legumes such as chickpeas and lentils balance the diet in more ways than one. They add fibre and trace elements, balance protein so less animal protein needs to be consumed and reduce the price of preparing meals.

There's a lot of discussion these days about whether high fat, high protein or high unrefined carbohydrates diets offer the best outcome for cholesterol management. The jury is still very much out on this. In the meantime the most natural programme for the management of cholesterol and heart health would surely be one in which food becomes your cardiovascular medicine. Each food listed in the "Protective Foods in Action" section has one or more helpful physiological actions. These include stimulating the heart muscle to pump blood more efficiently and help remove excess fluid, preventing platelet stickiness and thrombosis (clot formation), and supplying natural clot dissolving (fibrinolytic) substances. Some lower blood fats and thin the blood, allowing better circulation and improving bile flow and cholesterol excretion into the bowel. All the suggested foods are naturally high in nutrient density. A range of culinary herbs and spices, which are being increasingly studied for their amazing health benefits, are also included.

It's my advice to make these foods the basis of any dietary program aimed at preventing or reversing cardiovascular disease.

Just for starters, a glance through this range of protective foods should whet your appetite:

> onions, garlic, chives, leeks, spinach broccoli, kale, tomatoes, capsicums, green beans, pomegranate, blueberries, strawberries, raspberries, goji, olives, brussel sprouts, cabbage, bitter greens rocket/aragula, collards, ginger, turmeric, cinnamon, rosemary, thyme, oregano, parsley, coriander, fennel, mint, tarragon, sage, capers, all teas (especially green), cocoa, red wine, acai, quinoa, currants, horseradish, cauliflower, kiwi, kohlrabi, spinach, lemons, limes, oranges, grapefruit, beetroot, passionfruit, radish, asparagus, mango, pineapple.

Protective Foods in Action

Seafood

By eating certain fish two or three times a week you may be cutting your risk of heart disease by 50%. The omega-3 oils present in cold water fish like mackerel, herring, sardines, anchovy, tuna and wild salmon have a profound protective effect against heart disease and stroke. Fish and fish oils inhibit blood clot (thrombus) formation, protect arteries from damage and thin the blood. They lower triglycerides, small dense LDL-cholesterol and blood pressure and improve circulation to the extremities. At present it is not advised to eat large amounts of tuna because of the danger of mercury contamination.

Many people are still worried about consuming shellfish because they had the reputation of increasing cholesterol levels. All oysters, mussels, crabs, squid, lobsters, crayfish, prawns (shrimp) and clams have some cholesterol, but they also contain other cholesterol-type substances (called phytosterols) which tend to prevent any rise in blood cholesterol. With the possible exception of prawns, it's true to say that shellfish consumed as part of a low fat diet will generally lower LDL-cholesterol and triglycerides, while increasing HDL.

Pasture Fed Meat

Please see Chapter 7 for a discussion of the benefits of pasture fed verses grain fed meat.

Legumes/Beans

A cup of cooked dried beans every day will lower cholesterol, some say by around 20%. The cholesterol lowered is LDL, not HDL. Those maligned "chickpea eaters" of the Mediterranean were actually on to a good thing. Legumes and pulses are an often overlooked aspect of the Mediterranean diet.

Other examples of beans/legumes include lentils, kidney beans, green peas, baked beans, black beans, black-eyed beans, fava beans and soybeans. They all help control insulin and blood sugar levels.

It's been shown that soybeans raise the good HDL-cholesterol and actually help reverse the progression of coronary heat disease. All beans are useful to help counteract the effects of a high-fat diet when eaten at the same meal. Mexican "chilli", for example, mixes beans with meat and cheese. Or try huevos rancheros for a breakfast of eggs partnered with black bean puree and homemade salsa.

Remember to soak your legumes for at least 24 hours before cooking, ideally changing the soaking water a couple of times. Soaking removes most of the so-called "anti-nutrients" like phytates, making these foods easier to digest.

Nuts

Nuts and seeds (almonds, walnuts, sunflower seeds, sesame seeds, pine nuts, pumpkin seeds, chia, peanuts, etc.) are excellent sources of heart-healthy oils, which help manage cholesterol, by lowering LDL and particularly by raising the protective HDL cholesterol.

Nuts also offer some protection against blood clots. Their high arginine content helps reduce buildup of plaque in the arteries. Nuts contain high levels of "good" fats, particularly the monounsaturated and omega-3 types. Polyunsaturated oils are also best taken in the form of whole nuts and seeds, before they have been subjected to any manufacturing process. Nuts also naturally contain plant sterols, which are known to reduce cholesterol.

Nuts have been a staple food throughout human history. They can be perfectly stored in their shells, in which state they remain free from any form of degradation for a long time. Lots of nutrition in a safe, little package. But don't leave them processed and lying round in light and air. Same story as oils. They will oxidize and go rancid very quickly. Nor will they do the job covered in chocolate and sugar, or heavily salted. Some suspicion is also now falling on the temperature at which nuts are commercially roasted. This may involve extremely high temperatures, the effects of which are not yet understood. You can slow roast your own raw nuts at around 100C.

A small handful of nuts per day is more than adequate to reap the benefits and any more must be carefully monitored because of the high calorie content of nuts.

Eating almonds every day for at least a month has been shown to reduce cholesterol and lower other risk factors for heart disease. Two ounces of almonds also provides more than 50 per cent of your daily requirement of magnesium, a mineral that's essential for heart health. A dozen almonds with a small apple makes an ideal between-meal snack. Sprinkle chopped nuts and seeds onto salads or use them in baking, especially as a flour substitute in cookies and muffins, or a meat substitute in patties.

We suggest you limit your use of pre-ground nuts and seeds. Linseeds, for example, are particularly subject to easy oxidation, which makes flaxseed oils and ground food mixes somewhat risky. Better to grind freshly. If you buy nut oils, it's essential that they are fresh and have been stored in a cool, dark place. No guarantees, but do your best to obtain oils which have been cold pressed and stored in dark glass away from light and heat. Purchase in small containers that will be used in a shorter period of time.

Mixing nuts and seeds with herbs and spices (e.g. pesto) may be a traditional handy hint for minimizing oxidation. The antioxidants in the herbs and spices may lend protection to the oils in the nuts and seeds when emulsified by pounding in a mortar and pestle.

Oats

Oatmeal and oat bran can be as powerful as any cholesterol-lowering drug. Half a cup of oat bran per day is enough to lower LDL cholesterol by up to 20% over time. Unlike other grains, oats don't cause an increase in small LDL.

Oats can be eaten as oatmeal porridge or form the basis for making homemade bircher muesli. As a healthy snack, oatbran muffins can be consumed any time. Oatbran can be added to many foods, such as pancakes, rissoles, meatloaf, etc.

Oats are an excellent source of fiber, higher in protein than other grains like brown rice, they provide the type of complex carbohydrates which will maintain energy levels through the day. Oats help you cope with stress. They're also good for the healthy function of your thyroid, nerves and digestive system.

Unfortunately oats are more and more difficult to get in their whole state and are super-processed to facilitate fast cooking. Where possible, get the whole form, such as steel cut oats or grind your own. Soak overnight before cooking.

Avocados

Avocados have more protein than any other fruit. Sometimes known as "nature's butter", they have only about a quarter of the fat calories contained in the same weight of dairy butter. Ounce for ounce, they also provide more heart-healthy monounsaturated fat, vitamin E, folate, potassium and fibre than other fruits. They also exceed other fruits as a source of the powerful antioxidant lutein, which appears to protect arteries from hardening and the eyes from cataracts and macular degeneration.

You can mash avocado on wholemeal bread, into baked potatoes and even use it as a hydrating face mask. Avocado is an increasingly popular addition to green smoothies. It's one of nature's great "fast foods", making a meal out of any salad.

Eggplant

Eggplant may inhibit the rise of blood cholesterol that occurs after eating fatty foods such as cheese. Animal experiments have shown that even small quantities of eggplant can dramatically reduce the development of fatty plaques in animals. It works best if taken at the same time as foods containing fat or cholesterol.

Pomegranates

This dark red fruit is hot news these days as a very effective strategy for lowering LDL cholesterol and clearing out arterial plaque.

Pomegranates are packed full of disease-fighting antioxidants. Some studies suggest that they offer almost three times more than established antioxidant sources such as green tea, red wine, blueberry juice and cranberry juice. They also contain potassium, fibre, vitamin C and niacin, all of which contribute to increased energy and good health.

Pomegranates also increase the production of nitric oxide, which effectively relaxes blood vessels, allowing blood to flow more freely and protecting against plaque buildup in the artery walls. Researchers from the Vascular Surgery Clinic in Haifa, Israel, found that 50ml pomegranate juice per day over a 12 month trial period effectively reversed plaque buildup in a group of older subjects. Other studies have shown a reduction in plaque build-up of up to 44%. (1)

Apples

Could an apple a day keep the cardiologist away? Eating whole apples can lower the destructive LDL-cholesterol while maintaining or slightly elevating the protective HDL-cholesterol. This action is partly due to the high pectin content of apples. Whole apples suppress the appetite (an ideal situation for weight loss), cause a stable and prolonged rise in blood sugar rather than a rapid burst (good for type 2 diabetics) and lower blood pressure. They also lower the risk of stoke and heart attack.

Healthy people don't need to shy away from dried apples either, although care needs to be taken with levels of preservatives. Daily consumption of 75g dried apple (about 2 medium apples) has recently been shown to lower cholesterol in 160 post-menopausal women. After 6 months, LDL was down 24%. (2)

It's best to go for organic apples so you can happily eat the skin, where much of the nutritional value is stored.

Parsley

This common herb is a powerhouse of the nutrients that rejuvenate and detoxify. Include it when you make fresh juices. Nibble a few leaves when you want your breath to be sweeter. Chop it into salads, soups, sandwiches and pasta dishes. Parsley is also a stressbuster, and studies have shown it to be effective in reducing depression, lowering cholesterol and strengthening kidneys. Many herbalists recommend parsley to relieve the symptoms of rheumatism and PMS.

Cinnamon

This highly versatile ancient spice helps to relieve bloating and stabilize blood sugar. Cinnamon contains methylhydroxy chalcone polymer (MHCP), which speeds up the processing of sugar in your body. So putting cinnamon sticks in your tea, or sprinkling just a tiny amount on desserts, fruits, cereal and into smoothies, will make your insulin release much more efficient, which may slow ageing and help ward off diabetes and obesity which are part of the metabolic syndrome, a precursor to heart disease.

Artichokes

Artichokes are one of the best all-round foods for preventing arteriosclerosis. They are full of potassium and magnesium. Their cholesterol-lowering effect is the result of increased excretion of cholesterol in the bile and decreased intestinal reabsorption of the same excreted cholesterol, as well as the inhibition of cholesterol biosynthesis in the liver. The active agents responsible for this are mono- and di-caffeylquinic acids such as cynarin. Artichokes stabilize blood sugar and have a definite diuretic effect which may be of interest to those who tend to retain fluid.

Prepared artichokes are now widely available and make a tasty addition to most salads and casseroles. Both globe and Jerusalem artichokes are beneficial.

Mushrooms

Mushrooms are excellent for thinning the blood and helping to prevent heart attack and stroke. They are a good source of chromium, a natural cholesterol-lowering agent. Japanese Shiitake mushrooms help prevent the normal cholesterol-elevating effects of eating saturated fats. 60-90 grams of shiitake will actually reduce cholesterol associated with a moderate-fat meal. The Chinese black Mo-er mushroom (black tree fungus) commonly used in Szechuan and Mandarin cooking contains an active anti-coagulant molecule called adenosine. This substance acts in a similar fashion to aspirin by preventing platelet stickiness. See chapter 11 for more information on the therapeutic benefits of "functional" mushrooms.

Grapefruit

The active ingredient found in grapefruit's fibrous pulp is called pectin. The pectin of two grapefruit eaten each day will help increase the protective HDL-cholesterol while lowering total cholesterol. Over a period of time the active agents in grapefruit may help promote regression of atherosclerosis.

Caution: *People using pharmaceutical drugs should check whether grapefruit is contraindicated. In some cases grapefruit will change the metabolism of a drug, effectively leading to an overdose situation.*

Brown Rice

Rice fibre is as effective a cholesterol-lowering agent as oats and barley. Whole-grain brown rice is also an excellent food for lowering blood pressure. It is good for non-insulin dependent diabetics because it stabilizes blood sugar and insulin levels, and can form the basic cereal in any program aimed at weight reduction. The beneficial effects of eating whole grains are magnified by careful attention to chewing.

It's a good idea to keep some cooked whole grain such as brown rice on hand for adding to salads, rissoles, meat loaves, etc. Brown rice is perfect reheated for breakfast with the usual healthy accompaniments. Rice salad is an excellent choice for lunch. Use an olive oil vinaigrette or avocado/yoghurt dressing instead of mayonnaise (unless it's home-made). Additions can be as simple as a handful of chives and parsley from the garden. Try to include protein, such as a can of salmon, and some other cardioprotective foods such as onion, garlic, artichokes, capsicum or a range of chopped raw vegetables.

Fermented Foods and Probiotics

The consumption of probiotic-containing foods has drastically fallen over the last hundred years, or since the advent of refrigeration. It's a change that has huge implications, with which we are only just coming to grips.

Natural probiotics have been with the human race for hundreds of thousands of years and are vital for our health and wellbeing. When we are depleted of them through ingestion of chemicals, drugs or antibiotics, our health deteriorates.

Fermented foods like sauerkraut, kimchi, miso and tempeh are all examples of foods which take us back closer to the foods of our ancestors. Miso, tempeh and soya sauce are good examples of legumes that have been made more digestible through fermentation. Although legumes are an excellent food for most people, they are better fermented or at least extensively pre-soaked before cooking. These processes reduce dangerous lignans to which some people have an allergic-type reaction.

Garlic and the Allium Family

Garlic is probably best known for its antibiotic activity. However research continues to show that regular use will also lower blood pressure, reduce cholesterol and triglycerides and help dissolve clots. Aged garlic extract has been thoroughly tested for many decades, and is known to effectively inhibit the body's own production of cholesterol.

All members of the allium family (onions, leeks, chives, shallots, etc.) possess antioxidants containing sulphur. Chopping or crushing these foods produces allicin, a substance linked to decreased cholesterol production in the liver. Allicin is also a natural vasodilator.

In India food is not traditionally thickened with flour. Rather garlic is ground with ginger and onions and this provides the "body" for many dishes. Garlic and ginger may be peeled and combined in a food processor with a little water to form a paste, which is then lightly browned in oil or ghee. This mixture, together with other essentials of Indian cooking such as turmeric, coriander, cumin etc., forms a very healthy basis for Indian-style cooking. Beware the bottles of pre-cooked curry sauces in supermarkets. The added sugars, salt and thickening agents will not give you the same health advantages.

You can also slow roast unpeeled garlic cloves. A soft purée results, which can be easily squeezed out of the skin and is great to thicken sauces and casseroles. Add organic garlic to your own batch of healthy kimchi.

Ginger

The active substance in ginger is called gingerol. It's very similar in chemical structure to aspirin and acts in a similar way by preventing clots (thrombus formation).

A medical researcher in the US inadvertently discovered ginger to be an anti-clotting agent even more powerful than garlic or onions. He found that when he ate ginger marmalade for breakfast, samples of his blood platelets wouldn't stick together in laboratory experiments; nor did his blood coagulate as usual.

Turmeric

Turmeric contains the active substance, curcumin (5%), which lowers serum cholesterol by increasing bile flow (HDL-cholesterol actually rises) and inhibits platelet stickiness, making it an especially useful spice for those prone to thrombosis. As an added bonus turmeric is also an effective antioxidant, which can inhibit lipid peroxidation. Curcumin is now available in supplement form.

Chilli Peppers

Capsicum and chilli peppers are good fibrinolytic (clot dissolving) agents. Whole peppers, dry red pepper or pure capsaicin (the active hot pungent agent) have been known to lower cholesterol and triglycerides when taken in the presence of cholesterol-rich foods. The fibrinolytic activity of chillies is thought to be one of the main reasons why the Thai people experience so little thromboembolism. As clots start to form, the capsaicin in the chillies immediately gets to work to dissolved the potential clot. Peppers also naturally contain high levels of the anti-oxidants, beta-carotene and vitamin E.

Bananas

Monkeys may be wiser than we think. Their favorite food is among the most nutritious of tropical fruits. Fibre from green, unripe bananas reduces levels of the bad cholesterol and increases the good by as much as 30 per cent, while a ripe banana is one of the best ways to soothe an upset stomach. Bananas are a wonderful source of energy, can relieve heartburn and will also help decrease the risk of stroke. And with the possible exception of strawberries, no other fresh fruit is higher in minerals.

Seaweed

Seaweed is not just a superfood but also a food of the future. Most seaweeds contain around 70 essential minerals and trace elements. One of the best known seaweeds, the type used in Japanese miso soup, is wakame. Nori is the form used to make sushi. Both contain fucoxanthin, which has been shown to decrease LDL cholesterol and increase HDL. Seaweed also has a powerful effect on regulating triglyceride levels. Try to access seaweed harvested from non-polluted waters.

Coconut Oil and Water

Pure coconut oil contains lauric acid, which is a natural medium chain triglyceride and cholesterol stabilizer. High levels of medium chain fatty acids don't increase cholesterol.

Fresh coconut water is an excellent health tonic. It's high in minerals and electrolytes. Try coconut kefir as a non-dairy yoghurt alternative or use water kefir grains to lower the level of natural sugars and create an even healthier, naturally fermented and slightly fizzy drink from coconut water.

Unfortunately many commercial coconut milks and creams are sold in cans lined with bisphenol-A, a dangerous chemical, which can affect the nervous system. Acidic and fatty foods in particular can draw the chemical out of the lining of the can.

Coconut is so fashionable as to be almost a fad at the moment. It's best to consume it in moderation, especially if you don't live in a warm climate.

Fibre

Soluble fibre from beans and grains like oats helps reduce LDL and raise HDL. You will find beans in almost every ethnic diet, providing excellent sources of cholesterol-friendly fibre. Fibre is the natural food that keeps your microbiome (microorganisms in your GI tract) healthy.

Excellent sources of fibre include oats, chia, quinoa, broccoli, flax seeds, kiwi fruit and whole grains and legumes. Don't forget the brassica family, including cauliflower, cabbage and brussel sprouts, and also the onion family (onions, leeks, garlic, etc.).

Salt

Salt is not the problem most people think it is, as long as you are in control of your intake. This would be impossible if you rely on packaged or processed foods, which are high in salt. You can add 3-4 grams of salt daily if this is taken with a high fruit and vegetable diet (containing 3-4 grams potassium). The salt you add is then balanced. In any case deficiency of potassium, calcium and magnesium is more relevant to most forms of high blood pressure than salt per se.

Super Drinks

The current fashion for sugary drinks is said to be one of the main factors driving both the obesity epidemic and the sugar-linked rise in cholesterol. Adequate fluid intake is essential, particularly for those following a high fat and/or high protein diet. Here are some ideas for more healthy drinks.

Water

Inadequate water intake can cause cholesterol levels to rise, and making sure you drink enough water can help to lower cholesterol. Mineral waters are excellent, especially if they are high in magnesium and relatively low in sodium. Read The Watercure.com

Green Tea

Rich in flavonoids, it is a potent antioxidant, which lowers cholesterol and triglycerides while increasing the protective HDL. Importantly it prevents the oxidation of LDL.

Chai

Tea with the added phytochemical benefit of spices.

Green Drinks

Green vegetables are an absolute dietary must, but most people don't eat nearly enough. Green drinks can be the answer for some. They're high in soluble fibre, chlorophyll and magnesium with the benefit of antioxidants like beta-carotene and lycopene which protect against heart disease. Fresh from the garden, green vegetables provide enzymes and natural probiotics.

Unlike fruit juices, vegetable juices have a much more moderate effect on blood sugar.

Take advantage of the benefits of celery, spinach, cucumbers, parsley, kale, wheat grass and other sprouts, avocado, garlic, radish, cabbage, coriander and so on. Try adding spirulina or chlorella.

Use cabbage, broccoli and kale less frequently as these brassica vegetables can inhibit thyroid function, especially in their raw state.

Red Wine

Resveratrol is one of the best known antioxidants, and receives large amounts of publicity due to its presence in red wine. Resveratrol helps decrease oxidation of fats and is possibly linked with activating our longevity genes.

Watermelon Juice

Animals studies (Purdue University) have shown regular consumption of watermelon can significantly reduce the build-up of fatty acid deposits in the arteries. It is thought that the active ingredient responsible for this effect is citrulline.

Bone Soup

Don't waste good bones, especially from an organic or pasture fed animal. Heart healthy soup bases can be made from the bones of chicken, fish, beef, lamb, oxtail, duck, etc. Bone marrow is high in monounsaturated fats. Bone broth could almost be described as a type of alchemy. Prepare soup by long, slow cooking with the addition of a handful of herbs and a dash of cider vinegar or lemon juice—a little bit of acid helps release minerals from the bones. Minerals from the bones and phytonutrients from the herbs will all become more bioavailable through the process. Bone broth is an excellent aid to digestion.

Hot and Spicy Soup

The herbs and spices that Asian cultures add to bone soup are particularly healthy for heart and cholesterol protection. Benefit from the cholesterol-lowering properties of real stock infused with chili, ginger and garlic and other anti-inflammatory herbs like Thai basil and mint. Packaged stock and cubes may be too high in salt for those on a cardio-friendly diet.

Cabbage Soup

Cabbage is a great diet food, as many lovers of the cabbage soup diet have found. Cabbage helps lower cholesterol by preventing fat absorption after a meal. Red cabbage is high in antioxidants.

Naturally Fermented Beverages

It's not just boutique beer breweries which are currently enjoying a revival. Kefir and Kombucha are traditionally fermented drinks which are currently in vogue, as many people seek to improve their gut microbiome with the range of probiotics they contain. It's a topic that deserves to be approached with both enthusiasm and caution. I endorse this style of drink when produced with care and knowledge, however further discussion is beyond the scope of this book.

Chapter 10: What to Eat—Changing for the Better

When it comes to the evening meal, I'll leave it up to you. After reading this book you will know how to choose the best possible ingredients to put a meal together. It doesn't need to be complicated. The question of dinner can be solved simply with a generous serving of green, orange and red vegetables, together with various combinations of protein, pulses, nuts and seeds. Whenever you add a serving of wholegrains, keep to a half cup portion. If you use potatoes sometimes, once again keep the portion small and eat the skin. One or two small new potatoes or half a baked potato together with a larger serving of green vegetables is a more cardio-friendly balance.

With the wealth of online recipe resources now available, not to mention an abundance of excellent cookbooks, I don't intend to reinvent the wheel by filling these pages with recipes. A little knowledge is not always a dangerous thing. The more you learn about healthy foods and how they act as preventive medicine, the easier it will be for you to adjust your food preparation habits for the benefit and enjoyment of family and friends. If you want to read further, you could start by studying up on the Mediterranean diet.

Changing to Five Star Breakfasts

What's for breakfast? Many of us don't really feel confident about putting together a healthy breakfast.

Unfortunately most people are now addicted to starting the day with a sugar hit. Think breakfast cereals, fruit juice, toast with sweet toppings and sweetened hot drinks. To take care of your cholesterol, you may need to break old breakfast habits.

Earlier on we talked about how this whole cholesterol debate coincided with the development of packaged cereals, which were touted as the healthy alternative to a protein/fat breakfast like bacon and eggs. It's often said of such cereals that there is more goodness in the packaging than their contents. Yet the majority of us continue to eat these highly refined and excessively sweetened cereals. Fruit juice, that other favourite of everyday western breakfasts, is more likely than not a refined and highly sweetened beverage, with real fruit a minor ingredient. Even fresh fruit consumed as a large juice packs a blood sugar punch which is too high for good health.

This increased consumption of sugary breakfasts is a direct result of the scare campaign waged against fat-containing foods. What comes to mind when you think of eggs? Much maligned, eggs are in fact a superfood worthy of regular inclusion on the breakfast menu. Here are some other suggestions.

Superfoods for Breakfast

Berries, small apple or pear, grapefruit, pomegranates, goji berries, moderate serve of other whole fruit.

Eggs-boiled, poached or coddled are best-free range, organic.

Whey protein, kefir, yoghurt.

Nut and seed milks (better home made to avoid unnecessary polyunsaturated oils).

Vegetables-all green herbs, broccoli, onions, tomato, mushrooms, cucumber, avocado, kale, lacto-fermented vegetables, olives.

Naturally fermented cheeses like ricotta cheese and labaneh.

Whole grains, nuts, seeds. Nut butters.

Green tea or chai (may be sweetened with stevia). Freshly ground coffee.

Fish-kippers, herrings, sardines.

Some Breakfast Meal Suggestions

A note on breads

Labelling of bread is frequently misleading. Real "whole grain" is hard to find. Most bread is made from refined white flour with a few cosmetic additions mostly for marketing purposes. Many people now use a grain mill to make their own flour and bread. Artisanal breads like the heavy black rye favoured in northern Europe are a good choice.

Try the Toasting Test

One way to tell a good bread is to see how long it takes to toast. A longer time frame indicates a more stable product, with fewer AGEs being produced. *Don't eat burnt toast.*

Sweet smoothies—whey, berries and Greek yoghurt. Try adding coconut water, coconut kefir, nut butter or raw egg. No extra sugar needed, but use stevia if desired.

Green smoothies—blend green vegetables including herbs, spinach, kale, with avocado. You can also juice greens separately then blend with avocado. For more liquid try adding coconut water or mineral rich water. Add green powders like spirulina and barley greens.

Better juices—mainly vegetables like celery, spinach, cucumber and carrot, with some extras like apple, pineapple, ginger, lime segments. Avoid sugar spikes by adding a couple of tablespoons of soaked chia seeds and a slurp of coconut kefir or cream to fresh juice. Sip (or rather "chew") slowly over five or ten minutes.

Fresh fruit salad—half to 1 cup of fruit (leaning towards berries, apple and pear, rather than tropical fruit). Serve with plain Greek yoghurt and chopped nuts.

Summer tropical breakfast—sliced papaya with a squeeze of lime. Served with toasted coconut shreds and yoghurt or coconut kefir.

Homemade granola—toss whole rolled oats with chopped nuts and seeds in some orange juice, olive oil and a little honey. Slow bake on cookie tray at 100 degrees C for about 90 minutes, stirring occasionally, then increase temperature a little for another half hour.

Bircher muesli—soak mixture of whole grains, nuts, seeds, goji berries and cinnamon overnight in water to cover. Serve with yoghurt, kefir or cream, and fresh fruit.

Fridge Chia—overnight soak 3 tablespoons chia seeds, half to 1 cup water, half to 1 cup berries or cherries, 1 cup yoghurt/kefir/buttermilk, 2 tablespoons cream or coconut cream, a few chopped almonds. This makes 2 portions. Fine to keep for a couple of days.

Eggs Benedict (poached eggs with spinach)

Scrambled egg with smoked salmon and a side of greens like spinach or rocket.

Frittata: e.g. broccoli, green onion and goat cheese, but the possibilities are endless.

Breakfast Omelette—beat a couple of eggs with a fork, and maybe a dash of cream, milk or other liquid. Add some fresh herbs, spinach and/or finely chopped leftovers of your choice. Cook gently in a frypan.

Poached eggs with chorizo, spinach and spiced yoghurt.

Eggs lightly fried in a bell pepper ring. Serve with fried tomato.

Vegetable Hash—gently fry up leftovers like broccoli, cauliflower, onions, sweet potato, cooked quinoa. Add an egg or some bacon and a handful of fresh herbs.

Bacon, nitrate-free with spinach, mushrooms and grilled tomato.

Black bread with hummus, olives, fetta cheese, tomato, cucumber.

Crispbread with sardines or herring, tomatoes and red onions.

Sauteed mushrooms with chopped herbs and crème fraiche.

Avocado and tomato on toast.

Ricotta bakes—mix ricotta cheese with egg(s) and blueberries. Pour into individual muffin holders and bake at 180 degrees for 25 minutes. Blitz a punnet of strawberries to make a coulis (sauce).

Spinach and bacon pies—mix eggs with choice of spinach, bacon, prosciutto, onion, garlic, grated cheese. Bake about 30 minutes in individual muffin pans. For special brunches, cook the mixture in a base of filo pastry.

Buckwheat pancakes with sour cream and berries. Try a savoury version with Greek yoghurt, chopped hard-boiled eggs, chopped red onion, chives, fish roe.

Almond meal pancakes with garlic chives, chilli and bean sprouts.

Baked beans: Slow bake your own without added sugar. Freeze portions and defrost the night before needed. Serve with bacon, sausage or mushrooms.

Traditional Breakfasts

Sweet foods for breakfast have also drawn us away from our traditional roots, where breakfasts were much more savoury. Take a look at some of these ingredients from traditional breakfasts around the world. You'll get an idea of what we've lost and where you can possibly gain some inspiration for the changes you'd like to make. Perhaps your own ancestors ate this way?

Mediterranean: In many areas a Mediterranean breakfast still wouldn't feel right without a plate of olives. Even hotel buffet breakfasts in Turkey will always include a range of olives. Other traditional breakfast ingredients include leftover stone ground bread, olive oil, goat's milk, fruit, cheese, tomato, cucumber, onion.

Japan: Miso soup with tofu, seaweed, rice, fish, daikon radish, rolled omelette, ginger and other pickles.

Indonesia: Nasi campur (like a Balinese antipasta); fried rice, rice porridge, spicy chicken, hard boiled eggs, coconut vegetables, sambal

Scandinavia: Traditional soured cottage cheese, wholegrain rye bread, liver spread, pickled herrings, porridge with lingonberries, open-faced rye bread with lettuce, hardboiled eggs and fish roe, frittata with Jarlsberg cheese, bacon, leftover vegetables, potato pancakes with bacon and lingonberries.

UK: Kippers, back bacon, eggs, sausage, beans, mushrooms, fried onions, black pudding, bubble and squeak, fried or grilled oatcakes, porridge. In Wales they still eat laverbread, made from a mixture of oatmeal and seaweed puree, served with bacon and cockles. Laver is the same type of seaweed favored by the Japanese for making sushi (nori). Laver is a great source of vitamin A, C and folate, as well as omega-3 fatty acids and trace elements including iodine. It's often fermented too, making it an excellent probiotic food.

Vietnam: Borrowed the croissant from France but it's not what most eat for breakfast. A baguette is the legacy that has more currency. Not served with jam but a savoury filling including pickled vegetables, prawns, sausage, local pate, tomato or chilli sauce. Much more popular is pho (protein stock, slices or meat or chicken, herbs and spices, greens, rice noodles, chilli). From early morning you'll find a pho merchant's simmering cauldron set up every few metres along the footpaths in Vietnamese cities. A similar noodle dish popular for breakfast is called bun. Also a vermicelli noodle dish, it has more of a sour taste from the addition of tomato, mangosteen, lemon and lime. Dieters in Vietnam favour a breakfast made from cellophane noodles, usually made with a sour seafood broth with the addition fermented vegetables and eel.

Israel: Greek-style salad, omelettes and poached eggs, olives, yoghurt, fresh fruit, fish (especially herring), hummus, baba ganoush, labaneh (soft yoghurt cheese), bread.

Russia: Black bread, buckwheat porridge, sausage, yoghurt, buckwheat pancakes (blinis), curd cheese, fruit.

Himalayas: Tsampa made from ground roasted barley, yak butter and tea. This is a porridge with a difference. Barley fibre is an excellent prebiotic. It acidifies the lower bowel, down-regulates the production of cholesterol in the liver and increases bile production.

Lunches at Work and School

If you eat lunch out, we suggest you keep to grills, salads and soups (not canned). In most western cities we are spoilt for choice, and all that's required is our discrimination. Some cafes now offer excellent heavy bread options and will happily prepare you an open face sandwich of your choice. A wrap or sandwich can be OK but you may not want to eat all the bread. In Australia some cafes still make old-fashioned burgers—a good meal if you take to it with a knife and fork, skipping the bun and sauce. Fish and chip shops usually offer a grilled option and many sell a simple Greek salad as a healthy side. However perhaps you're one of the many who find eating out at lunchtime, especially in a healthy way, is both awkward and expensive.

Maybe you're also making school lunches for the family. Did you know that many western teenagers already have cholesterol/heart health profiles that put them well into the high risk category? Even though change is in the air, you'll be more than aware that many school canteens still frequently fail to provide and encourage healthy food choices. We can help our kids to care for their cholesterol by the examples we set, and the meals we serve them.

So let's get a little creative with making lunches using superfoods. Try, for example, foods that you would find on a tapas or antipasta platter. They make excellent lunch fare. Traditionally many of these are the leftovers of a previous meal, and can be delicious. Vegetable leftovers can be boosted with a can of seafood or hard-boiled egg. Meat leftovers can be turned into a great salad with a few raw vegetables and an olive oil and vinegar dressing. The varieties of "big salad" and Mediterranean salad are only limited by the imagination. Cold chicken and leftover frittata provide the basics for a good meal.

In winter, soup in a flask makes a welcome warm lunch. Add chopped leftovers to some meaty homemade stock together with some legumes and a big handful of fresh herbs.

A protein shake can come in handy at lunchtime. Delicious flavours are available, as well as sachets. Or you can carry a powered serving in a container that just needs the addition of milk or water. Make it a more filling meal with the addition of an apple and some almonds. Working women and teenagers find this a good choice, and it also works well in hot weather or whenever food might be inclined to spoil.

Dips are equally quick and easy. Keep the refrigerator stocked with raw celery sticks. Hummus and celery will keep you going surprisingly well. Make your own hummus varieties by adding various herbs or roasted, leftover vegetables. Works particularly well with beetroot.

A sandwich with fruit is still one of the easiest lunch foods. Wraps and mountain bread work well for children. Always use whole-grain, high fibre bread. There are advantages in choosing sourdough and many benefit from reducing or avoiding gluten grains. Breads now contain quinoa, pumpkin seeds and chia. The range of flours also offers more choice these days including buckwheat, spelt and many gluten-free options. Traditional heavy wholegrain rye bread, also known as black bread, is an excellent choice. The type of open face sandwiches that the Scandinavians prefer (one slice, not two), provide a better balance between carbohydrate, fat, protein and fresh vegetables.

Sandwich toppings such as those listed below may also be used as salads, dips and fillers for celery sticks, tomatoes, etc.

- lean, roast beef, mustard, watercress, red capsicum, mushrooms (layer)
- ricotta cheese, chopped celery, chopped apple, chopped walnuts (combine all ingredients)
- lettuce, pickled herrings, avocado, Spanish onion slices (layer)
- cottage cheese, chopped basil, chopped tomato, roasted pinenuts, chopped black olives (combine all ingredients)
- hummus, tabouli (on thin Mountain bread)
- red salmon, capers, chopped celery (mix with yogurt, lemon juice, Tabasco)
- small can sardines, 1 tablespoon mustard (mash with juice of a lemon).

Chapter 11: Nutritional Supplements to Help You Balance Your Cholesterol

Key Points

- Antioxidants are your best resource for protection against cholesterol damage.

- Antioxidants shouldn't be viewed in isolation—they work like an orchestra.

- Antioxidants are available in generous quantities from fruits and vegetables, and in particular, from herbs and spices.

Are You Suffering from Antioxidant Deficiency?

Most people are now familiar with terms like "antioxidant" and "free radical". Human beings, being oxygen breathing, are caught up in a cycle of using this oxygen for vital life processes, but then having to deal with potentially damaging by-products. Scientists say antioxidants "mop up" free radicals and that's a good analogy. Antioxidants, which the food chain bestows on us in abundance, protect us from the side effects of oxygen metabolism. They prevent, or at least slow down, oxidative damage.

However the 21st century food chain is something else again. We are living in a world with more free radicals and fewer antioxidants. Suffice to say that most foods, which have been grown in depleted soils and subject to storage, processing, radiation, etc. have very little left in the way of antioxidant activity. This presents a genuine danger to every aspect of human health.

Studies have shown that it's possible to protect and optimize cholesterol levels as well as prevent and even reverse heart disease with a synergistic approach using lifestyle choices and antioxidants. In *The Cholesterol Myth* I talked about having a high dietary intake of antioxidant nutrients such as vitamin E, vitamin C and beta-carotene to ensure optimal protection against the possible presence or formation of oxidized lipids and free radicals which we suspected were linked with the initial injury that could trigger off the destructive lesions of atherosclerosis. Some people were looking into selenium. But it was early days.

Nevertheless scientists were asking the right questions. Could low levels of antioxidants in the blood be associated with the increasing incidence of heart disease? Over many decades the *American Journal of Clinical Nutrition* (AJCN) has provided a wealth of information for interested professionals to keep up with the evolution of this field. Those who haven't kept up with this journal can find back issues free online.

For example, in 1987 a cross-sectional survey was published by AJCN, which looked at populations of middle-aged men in Scotland, Finland, northern Ireland, Switzerland and southern Italy. (1) Results showed that the more vitamin C you have in your cells, the less likely you are to die from a heart attack. In areas with the most heart disease, vitamin C levels were on average 33% lower and vitamin E levels around 25% lower. Since then research indicates that the same benefit applies for most antioxidants.

Important Antioxidants for the heart are:

Vitamin A, Lycopene, Lutein, CoEnzyme Q10, Zeaxanthin, Tocopherols, Tocotrienols, Selenium, CoEnzyme Q10, Flavonoids, Carotenoids, Polyphenolics, Resveratrol, Oligoproanthocyanidins, Catechins, Quercetin, Astaxanthin, Epigallocatechin, Epigallocatechin gallate, Vitamin C, Vitamin K.

One of the biggest changes since these early days is that we now understand that clinical studies looking into one or two single antioxidants were missing the point. This is why so many trials were reported to have failed. In fact many of the so-called "antioxidants" actually acted as oxidants under suitable physiological conditions. Others were not acting as antioxidants but as anti-inflammatory agents.

When we eat whole foods we get thousands of antioxidants/anti-inflammatory agents, not one or two. They form an orchestra or network of molecules that work synergistically and are involved in biochemical reactions involving electron transfer and also participate in other non-antioxidant-related biochemical reactions. For this reason large pharmacological doses of single antioxidants should be avoided in clinical trials. It would be safer and more effective to use whole extracts of foods containing families of antioxidants e.g. berries, fruit, vegetables and herbs which are high in a range of antioxidants which fall into categories known as mixed flavonoids, carotenoids, polyphenolics, tocopherols and tocotrientols.

These nutrient families have existed together in nature in various amounts and proportions for many thousands of years. Our bodies have evolved with a certain balance of these substances. This is why ethnic diets, such as the Mediterranean diet, continue to work so well. They allow for a positive transference of genetic material down through the ages, a process which appears to keep their respective communities healthy.

> Clinical studies looking into one or two antioxidants were missing the point and this is why so many trials were reported to have failed.

So when it comes to taking single antioxidant supplements, it's certainly possible to have too much of a good thing. It's a problem known as competitive inhibition. For example, a 30mg lycopene supplement is likely to compete with dietary lutein or a 20mg beta carotene supplement might compete with dietary lycopene. A lycopene supplement may block the positive effects of lutein against macular degeneration. A beta carotene supplement may interfere with the important role of dietary lycopene against prostate cancer. There is a similar story for retinol derivatives. Pharmacological doses of beta-carotene may actually act as an oxidizing agent in tissue such as the lung of a chronic smoker. So you can see why more and more experts are advising a diet high in fruit, vegetables, herbs and spices as the best source of antioxidants.

A diet based on this orchestra of food-based antioxidants and natural anti-inflammatory agents is one of the best ways of controlling and protecting lipoproteins. With knowledge, the supplemental extracts of such substances have the power to really improve your cholesterol profile—to increase the large fluffy LDLs and reduce the number of small density LDLs. The right supplements will also help to supercharge your HDLs and make them more efficient at removing cholesterol from blood vessel walls and controlling favourable cholesterol levels in general.

Tocotrienols—The New Take on Vitamin E

The first nutrition supplement that should be considered by those wishing to normalize lipoproteins is the new vitamin E complex of tocopherols and tocotrienols.

Many of the early clinical trials involving vitamin E were only looking at one particular form called "alpha tocopherol". We now know that the real vitamin E is actually a collection of 8 different molecules belonging to two categories. Four molecules (alpha, beta, gamma and delta) are called tocopherols and another four molecules with slightly different chemical structures are referred to as tocotrienols. They work together and their balance is of paramount importance in maintaining good health. This has been well illustrated by Dr Barry Tan from the American River Nutrition, Inc. who was the first to draw the attention of the nutrition industry to the importance of the tocotrienols/tocopherol balance.

Today we know that supplementation of diets with alpha-tocopherol reduces serum levels of both gamma- and delta-tocopherols in humans. Gamma-tocopherol enters the human brain without discrimination via the blood; however high alpha tocopherol in serum tends to suppress gamma-tocopherol in both serum and cerebrospinal fluid.

In human surgical tissues, there is an abundance of gamma-tocopherol compared to alpha-tocopherol. For example, the gamma-alpha ratios in adipose (31%), vein (33%), muscle (38%) and skin (53%) are much higher compared to those reported in plasma (typically about 10%). Smokers in 2 groups (Fijians and Cooks Islanders) have the same blood levels of alpha-tocopherol, but Fijians with twice the gamma-tocopherol levels have a 10 times lower incidence of lung cancer.

New understanding of this synergism and the dependence of the vitamin E family on each other tends to invalidate previous trials which used only alpha tocopherol and suggests they should be repeated with the full tocopherol/tocotrienol complex.

> The use of the vitamin E complex is the latest innovative approach to cholesterol balancing in the body.
>
> Evidence is growing for the powerful role of the tocotrienols in controlling cholesterol and reducing cardiovascular disease.

Human studies have shown that the tocotrienols have a huge impact on cardiovascular health and this is demonstrated by positive changes in serum lipids, including reduction in LDL cholesterol, reduction in oxidation of LDL and improvement in LDL receptor uptake, decreased cholesterol synthesis by down regulation of HMGCoA reductase, elevation in HDL cholesterol, reduction in hepatic triglyceride synthesis and VLDL secretion, reduction in serum levels of C-reactive protein (CRP), advanced glycation end products and expression of cell adhesion molecules.

The first study examining the effects of tocotrienols on cholesterol levels showed that total cholesterol could be reduced in the range from 5% to 35.9% and LDL cholesterol from 0.9% to 37% when 22 healthy volunteers took a capsule of palm oil-vitamin E each day for 30 days. The supplement contained 18mg tocopherols, 42mg tocotrienols and 240mg palm olein.

Similar changes were also noted in a longer 12 week double-blind trial involving 21 subjects with high blood cholesterol levels. Here total and LDL cholesterol were reduced 12 and 16% respectively when tocotrienols were added to a low fat, low cholesterol, alcohol free diet. High doses of alpha tocopherol supplements taken alone also lead to a depletion of plasma gamma tocopherol.

This is unfortunate when it is considered that alpha tocopherol has been routinely given to people for decades in order to reduce cardiovascular disease and gamma tocopherol is a major component in the prevention of heart disease. *The activity of alpha tocotrienol has also been shown to be 40 times higher than alpha tocopherol.*

Tocotrienols are also more potent scavengers of the harmful peroxyl radicals than alpha tocopherol and they give better protection against lipid peroxidation. This is important when we consider that oxidation of LDL cholesterol is known to be the first step in the development of atherosclerosis.

Many studies have shown that the tocotrienols exhibit antioxidant, antiproliferative, proapoptotic, antiangiogenic and anti-inflammatory activities. (2) (3)

Bergamot

As we know, most pharmaceutical products on the market succeed only in lowering total cholesterol, not just the bad guys. Bergamot, grown in the Calabrian region of southern Italy, is designed to increase the friendly HDL and decrease the small and dangerous LDL cholesterol levels while preventing oxidative damage to the lipoproteins.

In general people taking 500-1,000mg bergamot for 30 days may expect to experience:

- a decline in total cholesterol of around 23%
- a reduction in LDL of around 25%
- a reduction in triglycerides of around 28%
- an increase in HDL around 20%
- a decline in blood sugar of around 32%

    Mollace V et al. (4)

We have already covered the research which tells us that the large fluffy LDL particles are not damaging and in fact are important for carrying normal cholesterol to the body's cells for everyday use. The number of small LDL particles are the actual risk factors because these particles are more easily oxidized than the larger variety. The smaller particle size has a greater surface area compared to the large fluffy variety. Similarly not all HDL cholesterol is protective. This depends on HDL's capacity to move cholesterol from the blood vessel walls to the liver. This again depends on the HDL particle size and number, and other components of the HDL molecular structure.

Bergamot is one of the first of such innovative natural molecules to help balance the different types of cholesterol in the direction of good health.

The active components of bergamot are flavonoids. Melitidine and bruteridine have a statin-like action without the side effects. Naringin and neohesperidin lower harmful blood fats. Neoeriocitrin and rutin prevent oxidation of the LDL cholesterol, hesperitin reduces triglycerides and naringenin reduces blood sugar levels which is a bonus for people prone to diabetes.

In general people taking 500-1,000mg bergamot for 30 days may expect to experience a decline in total cholesterol of around 23%, LDL is reduced around 25%, triglycerides are reduced around 28% and HDL increases around 20%, Even blood sugar comes down around 32%. (4)

Pine Bark Extract

French Maritime Pine bark (Pinus pinaster) originates from the Mediterranean region. It is a hard, fast growing pine containing small seeds with large wings. It is a medium size tree with orange-red bark.

Maritime pine bark is rich in flavonoids and found to be among the most powerful natural antioxidants. Pine bark extract contains naturally-occurring phenolic compounds including proanthocyanidins, catechins and taxifolin.

Pine Bark extract (MPBE) at 200mg per day improves the integrity of the artery wall, increases arterial dilation by 32% and reduces oxidative stress levels.

Decreased vasodilation increases blood pressure in the arteries, which leads to an increased risk of heart attack, stroke and kidney failure. MPBE lowers blood sugar and improves vasodilation, two critical risk factors commonly found with high cholesterol and CVD.

Ubiquinol (Bioavailable Coenzyme Q10)

Ubiquinol is the reduced form of coenzyme Q10 and is a potent antioxidant present in LDL. It is absorbed about 4.5 times better than Coenzyme Q10. A single dose 100-200mg of ubiquinol increases blood levels 80-150% respectively within a 6 hour period. Increased plasma levels of ubiquinol increase the resistance of LDL to oxidation and reduce the levels of oxidized LDL. There is evidence that CoQ10 influences gene expression leading to a reduction of LDL.

Long term supplementation with 300mg per day causes a 4 fold enrichment in ubiquinol in the plasma and each LDL particle gains 2.8 ubiquinol molecules. These together with the tocopherol/tocotrienol complex, form the major barrier in preventing LDL and HDL oxidation. The rate of lipid oxidation increases markedly with the disappearance of ubiquinol.

In addition, low levels of ubiquinol are linked to cardiovascular inflammation. In fact depletion of ubiquinol in the blood is a marker of oxidized or damaged LDL. Plaque formation is characterized by inflammation, which attracts immune cells to the damaged LDL particles.

Pantethine (B5)

Pantethine is an active stable form of vitamin B5. It consists of 2 pantothenic acid molecules joined together by 2 sulphur atoms. These 2 sulphur atoms are part of the active component known as cysteamine and cystamine when pantethine is metabolized.

While the exact mechanism of action of pantethine is not known it is thought that it involves several enzymes involved with cholesterol synthesis. It also helps to convert fat to energy.

Oral supplementation with pantethine (900mg/day) results in decreases in total cholesterol, triglycerides, LDL cholesterol, Apo-B100 and an increase in HDL cholesterol and Apo(A). Results may not be seen until about 4 months of use.

Policosonal

Policosonal was originally portrayed as a natural cholesterol-lowering dietary supplement. A natural anti-oxidant and anti-inflammatory agent, it lowers total and LDL cholesterol without side effects while at the same time elevating HDL. It was thought to inhibit abnormal platelet aggregation as well as the formation of lesions in the arteries. Research shows that it dramatically lowers LDL and raises HDL up to 29% at a dose of between 5 and 20mg/day.

More recently the initial Cuban trials, which were conducted with Cuban sugar cane policosanol, were repeated by five different research teams from around the world. These well-designed trials used both Cuban and non-Cuban policosanol products. None of the trials outside Cuba have been able to confirm the lipid-lowering activity of policosanol. At this stage policosanol should not be looked at as a cholesterol-lowering agent. (5) (6)

Curcumin—Improving the Action of LDL Receptors

So if active viable LDL receptors are an important aspect of protection against heart disease how can you improve the integrity and activity of what might otherwise be sluggish LDL receptors? One interesting way to achieve this may be to turn to the ingredients in an Indian curry, especially turmeric.

The active component in turmeric is a yellow pigment called curcumin. This substance constitutes 3-5 % of the herb but has recently been isolated and used as a powerful anti-inflammatory agent. Working on many mechanisms in the body, it is able to inhibit most inflammation promoting mediators such as C-reactive protein and cytokines and has been shown to be comparable to potent drugs such as hydrocortisone and non steroidal anti-inflammatory agents.

Curcumin is a powerful antioxidant, powerful enough to reduce the oxidation of cholesterol. Indian research has shown that when 10 healthy volunteers consumed 500 mg of curcumin per day for 7 days, not only did their blood levels of oxidized cholesterol drop by 33%, but their total cholesterol dropped 11.63%, and their HDL (good cholesterol) increased by 29%. (7)

How does curcumin work? Curcumin lowers total cholesterol by cranking up the genes in the liver, which increase the production of proteins required to make LDL receptors. The other interesting aspect of the curcumin treatment was that it increased the production of bile acids and thus the ability to lower levels of cholesterol while stimulating the bile flow.

These results were confirmed in 2007 by a German group who also found a seven fold upregulation of the genetic material required for LDL receptor manufacture using curcuminoid pigments. (8)

In another example, Chinese workers published data the following year to show that curcumin increased the genetic expression of the genes that make protein for the LDL receptor and concluded by saying "These findings contribute to our further understanding of the cholesterol-lowering and anti-atherosclerotic effects of curcumin". (9)

Medicinal Herbs and Ethnopharmacology

There are many herbs that can elicit blood vessel toning, blood purifying, anti-platelet, cholesterol lowering, cardiac stimulating and blood pressure normalizing effects.

Herbs were our original "pharmacy". Evidence of their use goes back as far as 5000 years. They are still used extensively in societies which maintain a strong connection to traditional medicine. Culinary herbs and spices form part of this family of active natural substances with beneficial effects on metabolism and health that are being increasingly well documented.

Garlic

Garlic is one of the world's best researched herbs. It's a great antioxidant and high in organosulphur compounds which protect against free radical damage.

Garlic, together with onion, has been extensively researched in India, where it is the staple of much Indian cooking. Some Indians abstain from garlic and onions for religious reasons, but otherwise eat the same diet, thus creating an ideal research sample. Those who abstain were found to have significantly less favorable lipid profiles, compared to those who ate the most garlic and onion.

Over the last 30 years, a well-known supplement known as Kyolic Aged Garlic has been subject to hundreds of tests which have indicated its value in lowering LDL cholesterol, raising HDL and preventing LDL oxidation. Kyolic has also been tested for safety of use in conjunction with statin drugs and warfarin. (10)

Hawthorn

Hawthorn berries are powerful antioxidants, rich in bioflavonoids. Hawthorn tonic has been used for centuries in Europe as a general heart tonic. Hawthorn increases blood flow and oxygen to the heart, and strengthens the heart muscle. It also lowers LDL and triglycerides.

Gugulipid

This is a standardized extract from the Indain myrrh tree, which has also been shown to lower triglycerides and cholesterol. It increases the body's natural ability to metabolize cholesterol in the liver. (11)

Fenugreek

Fenugreek seeds are included in many Indian spice blends, and as such are often consumed on a daily basis. They contain a natural substance similar to guar gum, which is known to reduce total cholesterol, LDL, VLDL and triglycerides without lowering the beneficial HDL cholesterol. Fenugreek is an important source of diosgenin, which is included in many natural products because of its beneficial effects on cholesterol metabolism.

Gingko

Gingko biloba is an excellent antioxidant. It has a powerful modulating effect on the circulating system, particularly the blood vessels supplying the brain. Gingko dilates blood vessels to give increased blood flow, while enhancing cellular energy production in the brain. It also inhibits the harmful effects of free radicals and platelet aggregation, and hence tends to prevent thrombosis.

Developing senile dementia is a worry for many of us as we age. It's not the same thing as Alzheimer's Disease, where specific neurones begin to deteriorate and die. Some forms of dementia are linked to hardening of the arteries leading to the brain. Thus vascular insufficiency (reduced blood flow to the brain) is frequently a major factor in age-related cerebral disorders. Gingko is particularly useful for the prevention of "mini-strokes" (transient ischaemic attacks or TIAs) as well as a large variety of non-haemorrhagic strokes (the types resulting from a clot, not a haemorrhage) due to its potent inhibition of platelet aggregation.

Functional Mushrooms

Mushroom extracts have been widely used for medicinal purposes in Asia for thousands of years. Excretion of cholesterol in the stool has been observed with ingestion of mushroom fibre. Shiitake mushroom, which figures prominently in the traditional diet of long-living Okinawans, is high in cholesterol-lowering beta glucans and also in a rare beneficial polysaccharide called lentinan, which has also been shown to lower cholesterol. Shiitake mushrooms are high in manganese, selenium and zinc as well as a number of phytonutrients which have antioxidant and immune-regulating properties. Research on oyster mushrooms also indicates the importance of mushroom sterols in the reduction of cholesterol absorption by competitive inhibition. (12) (13)

Other Vitamin and Mineral Supplements

Magnesium

Extremely beneficial for all aspects of heart function. Improves lipoprotein balance and helps reduce platelet stickiness.

Western populations are frequently low in magnesium. Found in nuts and greens, dietary sources are usually inadequate. Water can be a good source, but only in certain areas. Many common pharmaceutical drugs deplete magnesium, including those used to manage cholesterol. So does stress and the social drugs we use to manage it, like coffee and alcohol.

Seek professional advice on the best type and dose of magnesium for you.

Vitamin C

Did you know that animals can make their own vitamin C, but humans can't? What's more, western diets are generally low to inadequate in vitamin C, which is a major antioxidant and essential to most biochemical reactions in the body including the repair and stabilization of blood vessel walls. Lack of vitamin C can signal the body to look for other means of repair, such as creating more cholesterol.

The B Vitamins

A good B complex for heart health will particularly include vitamins B1, B3, B5, B12, folate and B6.

Niacin (B3)

We haven't heard the last of this one, even though it's been knocked off the scene by the statins. Niacin has been around for more than 50 years, but hasn't gone very far in a marketing sense, probably because it's not a drug. It's not widely prescribed, however it is still a very effective cholesterol-lowering agent, while at the same time raising HDL. Niacin came to fame when it was the only cholesterol-lowering agent found to reduce the death rate in the Coronary Drug Project. Researchers are still debating the combination of niacin with statin drugs, but there's a strong argument for it because statins have no success with raising the protective HDL cholesterol, whereas this is a strength of niacin.

You can find niacin in foods including white meats, organ meats, peanuts, yeast and some types of fish but the amount used to lower cholesterol is considerably higher. Get advice before taking supplemental niacin as it can cause side effects including skin flushing. Liver function also needs to be monitored. It may not be suitable for everyone.

Vitamin K

Vitamin K is helpful for cholesterol management at the right level, but not in excess. Eat plenty of greens. The highest food source of vitamin K2 is natto. Those who can cultivate the taste for this unusual food will receive protection against high cholesterol and stroke. Supplementation with vitamin K needs to be monitored by an expert.

Glutathione (GSH)

Glutathione helps prevent oxidation of LDL. It is one of the body's important antioxidants. Glutathione levels are increased by consuming whey protein and high quality fresh vegetables and protein. Curcumin enhances glutathione metabolism. Exercise and stress reduction are also essential.

Taurine

Taurine lowers LDL and can significantly increase HDL. It's an amino acid that also increases gall bladder function.

Arginine

Arginine helps keep your blood vessels clean by breaking down plaque. It improves circulation by relaxing blood pressure and increasing nitric oxide. This research won the Nobel Prize.

In people with heart and vessel disease, L-arginine restores production of nitric oxide and improves blood flow and in so doing relieves symptoms of heart and vessel disease. (14).

Carnitine

L-Carnitine also lowers LDL and increases HDL. It occurs naturally in protein-rich foods, plus avocado, asparagus and peanuts. Get advice from your health practitioner on its use in supplementary form.

Lysine

Lysine (together with vitamin C and proline) has been used to lower levels of lipoprotein (a), a major independent risk factor for cardiovascular disease.

Tailor Your Cholesterol Care Plan

Many factors will determine which supplements will be best for you. Price will be a factor but most importantly, biochemical individuality needs to be taken into account. We suggest you obtain the guidance of a medical professional with expertise in clinical nutrition to tailor your personal cholesterol plan.

Here's an example of a program put together for one patient who needed to normalize cholesterol and triglyceride levels, reduce blood pressure and inflammation, and reverse or slow down a tendency towards oxidation of proteins and fats.

- Ubiquinol 150mg twice daily
- Tocotrienol/tocopherol 250mg twice daily
- Bergamot 500mg twice daily
- Pantethine 450mg twice daily
- Curcumin 500mg twice daily
- Niacin 500mg twice daily (increase dose slowly to minimise flushing)
- L-lysine plus vitamin C (60mg) 1g twice daily
- Magnesium citrate (150mg elemental Mg) twice daily
- Omega-3 fish oil 2g twice daily.

Chapter 12: Exercise and Stress Management— More Important than Ever

Key Points

- Exercise is essential. Find out what you enjoy and do it regularly.
- Stress and negative emotions are bad for your heart and cholesterol.
- Meditation and stress management techniques are as effective as any other approach to cardiovascular health.
- Optimism, happiness and life satisfaction contribute to a healthy heart.
- Kindness, touch and social support all benefit heart health.
- "Cynical hostility" is the worst personality profile for heart health.

In my clinic in Sydney I have seen many patients presenting with various forms of cardiovascular disease over the last 35 years. Imminent heart attack or stroke usually prove to be a potent motivating factor and compliance with dietary and lifestyle changes is usually good.

Exercise

Let's firstly look at exercise in the context of cholesterol management and cardiovascular health.

Regular exercise reduces many of the established risk factors for heart disease. Lounge lizards have the same risk for heart disease as people with high blood pressure, abnormal blood lipids, obesity or a history of smoking.

Exercise promotes general good health by leading to weight reduction, lower blood pressure, a better profile for both blood lipids and blood sugars, as well as improved insulin sensitivity. Swimming and running have been shown to help metabolize the stress hormone, adrenaline. It's even been claimed in one scientific study that patients with newly diagnosed heart disease, who participated in a formal exercise program, reduced their death rate by 20-25%. (1)

Moderate Daily Exercise

A good exercise program improves the body's utilization of oxygen. This leads to better muscle function. We sometimes forget that our heart is a muscle too. When muscles perform with less fatigue we build stamina.

Regular exercise also improves the function of muscles in the blood vessel walls by enhancing the capacity of blood vessels to dilate and take in a good supply of oxygen. This, in turn, improves muscle strength, flexibility and bone health, which reduces many types of physical disability.

You don't need to start running marathons to reap the benefits of exercise. Thirty minutes of moderate exercise daily is generally considered adequate for most people. This can be achieved by brisk walking at about 5 km/hour. You might also enjoy activities like swimming, cycling, dancing, rebounding, tai chi, yoga or going to the gym. Just working around the house or yard can improve fitness. Activity can also be intermittent, say 3 bursts of 10 minutes during the day, and include activities like taking the stairs instead of taking the lift, or walking to the corner shop for a forgotten item instead of driving. Taking public transport also results in a lot of incidental exercise compared to always using the car. In fact one research study which looked at over 6000 men over a six year period found that the best heart fitness results and lowest death rates were found in individuals who started out with the lowest fitness rates but made some real effort over the period. (2)

However, generally speaking, adults who are the least fit have a mortality risk that can be up to five times higher than the most fit.

Exercise Safety

Even if you have had a previous heart attack, bypass surgery, angioplasty or stent insertion, exercise is still very important. It's always advisable to get medical approval when planning your exercise program.

A common question from people with a history of or high risk profile for cardiovascular disease, concerns the safety of exercise. That's understandable. Many have had the experience where exertion resulted in adverse symptoms just before a heart attack.

It may be reassuring to note that 90% of heart attacks occur at rest, not as the result of physical exertion. It takes 400-800,000 hours of exercise before one person experiences a cardiac event. Those with existing heart disease who do not exercise are at higher risk of experiencing an event. In this case it is once in every 62,000 hours. (3)

It's sobering to realize that an inactive person's risk of a heart attack is almost 50 times higher than the person who exercises 5 times a week. (3)

So before you start on any exercise program make sure you're comfortable by exercising in loose clothing and wearing appropriate footwear. Before commencing your workout, always warm up with stretching or gentle movement. Similarly, spend some time cooling down when you have completed your activity. Just slowing the pace towards the end of your activity will largely achieve this.

Warning Symptoms During Exercise

If you feel at all unwell during exercise you should take a rest immediately. Warning symptoms include dizziness or lightheadedness, chest pain (including pain or pressure in the chest), jaw or neck pain (possibly extending into the shoulder, back or arm), shortness of breath, irregular heart beats (e.g sensations of the heart skipping beats, palpitations or thumping), gas pains or indigestion, excessive sweating, loss of colour or nausea. These symptoms should be discussed with your doctor as soon as possible.

Some activities may be off limits. These include weights and other heavy lifting, mowing, shoveling earth or snow, scrubbing, etc. Challenging hills needed to be approached with caution while walking. Isometric exercises such as push-ups and sit-ups may be too much to start. Lighter aerobic sets of exercise are usually better. If the program has been discontinued for several days due to a vacation, illness or bad weather, it is always good to ease yourself slowly back into your routine. Never push yourself to achieve certain times and heart rates. You may need to rethink your idea about "personal best".

Hidden dehydration can be a problem. If you exercise outdoors always drink plenty of water even if you don't feel thirsty. Be mindful of temperature changes. If it is too hot, too cold or humid, you may get exhausted more quickly. Extreme temperatures can increase the workload of your heart.

More detailed information concerning exercise programs for those with cardiovascular concerns can be obtained from the Australian Heart Foundation website. (4)

How Exercise Helps Keep Cholesterol Healthy

We talked earlier about how important it is to reduce the dangerous small dense LDLs and increase the lighter fluffy LDLs. Exercise is another way to do this.

To give you an example, when 13 men around 47 years of age were put on a 14 week endurance-oriented exercise training program, their calculated LDL levels remained the same. However, on closer examination it was found that the chemical composition of the LDLs had changed after exercise. There was an increase in the fatty substances in the LDL (like cholesterol and phospholipids) which resulted in the small dense variety turning into the healthy, lighter LDLs. At the same time the men also lost fat mass around their waists and their blood triglyceride, insulin and glucose levels all came down towards normal.

This finding indicates that cholesterol, rather than being a risk factor, was highly beneficial because of its ability to enrich and change the shape and chemical composition of the LDLs, making them more cardioprotective. (5)

Research into the benefits of running reveals similar results. When 12 long-distance runners were compared with 64 sedentary men it was found that the runners had lower levels of small dense LDL and higher levels of the healthy HDL fractions. (6) However, as we said before, you don't need to take up running.

Take note of the results of a recent Japanese study involving 30 men and women (aged 64 years) with high blood fats. This study focused on the effects of increasing moderate physical activity over a 6 month period.

The results showed that even this moderate amount of exercise was able to significantly increase the particle size of the LDLs, which rendered them less susceptible to oxidation and hence atherogenic potential. This is one of the first studies on physical activity to demonstrate cross talk between small dense LDL and oxidative stress. It showed "that the concomitant changes in small dense LDL and oxidative stress can be associated with the reduction of the development of cardiovascular disease, even when there is a moderate increase in physical activity among hyperlipidaemic subjects".(7)

A word of caution for statin users

If you wish to embark on an exercise program to lower your cholesterol level please see your doctor first. Your doctor should be aware that statin use presents another obstacle to the fitness ambitions of cardiovascular patients.

Research has recently drawn attention to the possible muscular side effects and impairment of mitochondrial function of the statins. One group decided to study the effect on muscle fitness in 37 sedentary overweight or obese adults who were randomised over a 12 week period to either aerobic exercise training or a combination of exercise training while taking the statin drug, simvastatin (Zocor).

The results were interesting because cardiovascular fitness increased by 10% in the exercise only group but increased just 1% in the group who also took the statin drug. Skeletal mitochondrial function also decreased in the statin group as demonstrated by a decrease in the activity of a key mitochondrial enzyme (citrate synthase) by 4.5%. The exercise only group showed an increase in activity in this enzyme of 13%. (8)

Exercise training has also been shown to have other specific cardiovascular benefits, such as helping to dissolve any unwanted clots (thrombi) in blood vessels. Normally when these form, the body is able to dissolve them by a process called fibrinolysis. Acute clinical events resulting from hardened arteries (such as myocardial infarction and stroke) are associated with impaired fibrinolysis.

Intermittent claudication is another related condition which causes pain in the legs due to a narrowing or blockage to the main artery of the leg. Fibrinolysis is impaired. After 6 months of treadmill exercise training, 21 men with intermittent claudication experienced significant improvement. This was shown as a 23% decrease in the enzyme which normally blocks the breakdown of clots and a 28% increase in the enzyme which activates their breakdown. (9)

Stress Management

For optimal cardiovascular health, lowering your stress level is equally important to keeping fit and active . Everyone is subject to some degree of unwanted stress and we can all benefit from keeping it in check.

I've found that there's a subgroup of patients who are fit and eat well, but simply don't achieve much benefit from minimizing the usual risk factors for cardiovascular disease. Nor does the problem appear to be genetic. Yet there is one factor which all appear to have in common. They complain of stress. They are often frustrated or angry with life and find it difficult to communicate their problems in emotionally healthy ways.

It used to be fashionable to talk about these people as "A type" personalities. Key traits included free-floating hostility, aggressiveness, competitiveness, a constant sense of urgency, impatience, constant striving for ill-defined goals, cynicism and fast, abrupt patterns of speech and movement. Think Basil Fawlty.

Fear and anxiety are the other two emotions that can cause us problems, and can afflict other "types" as well. We now understand more about the highly sensitive personality types who are tuned into the slightest stress to the point of being in a state of chronic hyperarousal. This state is linked to chronically high levels of adrenaline and other stress hormones as well as cortisol, a marker of chronic stress.

Whatever the cause, chronic sympathetic nervous system overstimulation has been linked with chronic, elevated cholesterol levels. For example, Argentinian air force pilots under prolonged emotional stress during the Falklands' war were found to have significant elevation of urinary adrenaline and plasma cholesterol levels. Other research has found these emotional states linked with increased triglycerides and the mobilization of fatty acids into the blood. Put this together with the reduction in antioxidant levels which are used up by the higher demands of emotional stress.

We have also entrenched many stress-linked behaviors into cultural normality. Workaholism is a good example. The concept of "soldier on" is endemic.

Dealing with Anger and other Negative Emotions

Should you rant, rave and bash pillows? Or quietly smoulder, while the resentments undermine your endocrine system?

Basically the best way of dealing with any negative emotion is to nip it in the bud right at the outset. Don't let angry outbursts grow into the type of chronic anger which can constrict the blood flow of your large blood vessels, increase your blood pressure and increase your risk of heart attack or stroke.

Some years ago "behavior modification" was all the rage, as research showed that it successfully reduced the time urgency and hostility components of the type A personality. There were many techniques being explored, from wearing rings that relied on skin resistance to indicate emotional states, to making a toy train roll around a track by controlling thoughts and emotions.

These days there's more interest in "cognitive behavior therapy" and anger management classes, but the aim is the same. Now in conjunction with a trained practitioner we can learn to acknowledge (rather than repress) our difficult emotions and acquire tools for changing these entrenched emotional habits. Ideally the change comes simply from the observation and acknowledgement of the emotion, rather than adding more stress through attempts to consciously change. It's more about learning to let go. The emotion arises, we see it, feel it, possibly we name but we don't feed it. We don't encourage it. We may be taught to sit with the feeling of discomfort till it dissipates, or return our thoughts to a neutral, peaceful space. We learn to relax away from impulsive behaviours.

Meditative Practices

If this sounds like a meditation practice, that's no coincidence. I've been recommending some form of meditation, "calm" or "listening" practice for many decades. The research had become compelling. For example, Professor James Lynch from the Psychophysiological Clinic and Laboratories at the University of Maryland School of Medicine showed us long ago that when people talk their blood pressure rises and when they listen it subsides. (10) (See Figure 5 below.) Sounds like something the Chinese have known for millennia. Big talkers are prone to heart attack. Incessant talking is linked to hypertension while listening induces the opposite state, although according to musicologist Don Campbell, that depends on your choice of music.

Figure 5: The Effect of Talking on Blood Pressure
(Systolic BP-top line and Diastolic BP-lower line)

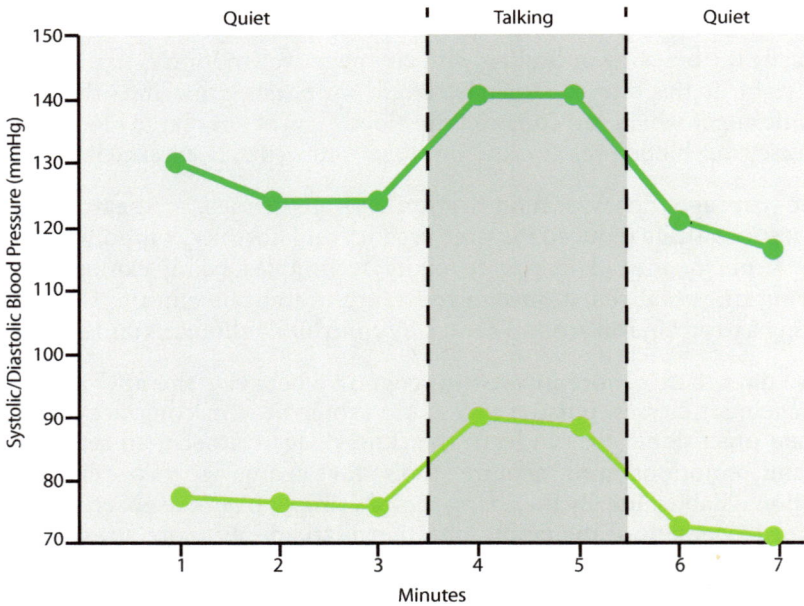

I was also impressed by the early research results of scientists studying a technique called Transcendental Meditation (TM). A typical study analyzing the health insurance statistics of 2000 people practicing TM over a 5 year period showed that the meditators had 87% less hospitalization for heart disease, 55% less for cancer, 87% less for nervous system disorders and 73% less for nose, throat and lung problems in all of the TM practitioners. There were also markedly fewer incidences of illness in 17 medical treatment categories and less than half the doctor visits irrespective of their diet and daily exercise patterns.

The TM researchers undertook one study to examine the possibility that meditation might help lower cholesterol. Subjects practiced meditation (or control) for almost a year. Those in the meditation group experienced falls in cholesterol between 5 and 35%. This is most likely due to a drop in the chronic stress hormone, cortisol, and thus a drop in the precursor molecule, cholesterol.

TM meditation was also shown to have beneficial effects on patients suffering from angina pectoris. Meditators also produce less adrenaline (epinephrine), which has a beneficial effect on the tone of the heart muscle, blood pressure and exercise tolerance.

Dr Herbert Benson was the first to take the TM research and produce his own medically tested relaxation program for the mainstream—*The Relaxation Response* (11). He basically just replaced the Sanskrit mantra with the word "one" while following the same general technique. This helped remove the cultural strangeness which many found to be an obstacle.

We've come a long way since then. Now it's medical mainstream in some US hospitals to offer courses in what has become known as "mindfulness-based stress reduction" (MBSR). You are taught how to catch your own stress reactions as they arise, more difficult than it may sound. You are also taught the skills of being mindful. It's just like going to the gym. There are brain circuits and awareness patterns you need to build, like how to ground yourself in the awareness of your body; like how to return to the feeling of your own breath, which is a very cheap, effective and portable stress management tool once you get the hang of it.

There are now literally thousands of books to educate those interested in this field. In our clinic we recommend books by Eckhart Tolle, Thich Nhat Hahn, Joan Borysenko and Jon Kabat-Zinn to those who show interest. Websites and apps also abound. Dr Rick Hanson's Just One Minute is an excellent resource, also available online.

The increase in the practice of yoga in the west over the last 20 years has also exposed many people to the benefits of a meditative practice. Anything that requires your full attention and takes you away from nagging stressful thought patterns helps break the stress cycle. Pottery and gardening are two good examples. And if you have an addiction to "shock jock" media, consider working on that one too. You have plenty of your own stress to practice on without also sucking it in from the airways.

Human Emotions: The Lifestyle Heart Trial

Over 30 years ago a landmark cardiac study was published in the Lancet that many found very exciting at the time. Dr Dean Ornish and colleagues showed for the first time that lifestyle changes could lower cholesterol and actually reverse heart disease. Using a combination of a low-fat vegetarian diet, moderate aerobic exercise, stress-management training and social support they were able to reverse blockages in coronary arteries in 28 patients. Dr Ornish has stayed on centre stage in the diet debate which has raged over this time as to whether a high or low fat diet is the more healthy choice.

The diet was very effective in lowering cholesterol and achieving all the other cardio targets it set out to achieve. It was also very restrictive and did not take advantage of the current knowledge of how certain foods can decrease cardiovascular risk. Things like olive oil, eggplant, red wine etc. Assumed risk probably eliminated many whole foods that are not dangerous. No coffee, no alcohol, not much in the way of Mediterranean joie de vivre. But here we should ask ourselves about the non-tangibles that may have made the Lifestyle Heart Trial work. The patients were taught to meditate and practiced for an hour a day. They also had support group meetings twice a week with a clinical psychologist who taught communication skills and encouraged the sharing of emotions.

According to Dr Ornish "underneath their differences they, almost to a person, felt a sense of isolation from parts of themselves and their own feelings, isolation from other people and isolation from a higher force, whatever that meant to them. And I came to see that that is where chronic stress that leads to illnesses like heart disease begins. It's that perception of isolation and alienation" (12). He saw this sense of isolation as being the root cause of personality traits like cynicism, hostility and self-involvement. These have been shown to be linked to cardiovascular risk. Because of this observation he changed the focus of the group more towards these intangibles.

Optimism and Positive Psychology

My practice is located in Sydney. For over 10 years Sydney has hosted an international conference on the benefits of positive psychology. The conference titles vary from time to time, probably to extend their reach, but mostly they go by the title, "Mind and Its Potential".

Delegates number in their thousands, and include many health practitioners. Many key international speakers on this circuit are also attracted, including Dr Martin Seligman, whose book *Learned Optimism* probably started the ball rolling over 30 years ago.

Even though you'd hardly call it a mainstream, "mindfulness" has become a key focus of many psychological practices in Sydney. "Happiness" is being explored in all its possible manifestations. We're the home of interesting characters like a clinical psychologist who goes by the name of Dr Happy and a medical doctor psychotherapist, Big Shakti. There are many professionals like these who keep things moving along while the double-blind crossover experts try to figure out what their approach should be.

Most recently on this subject, researchers Julia Boehm and Laura Kubzansky from Harvard have drawn a lot of media attention with their review of over 200 studies, which actually have looked at psychological wellbeing and heart health. It's good to get this information out there, even if the whys and wherefores are still getting sorted and the key points within a disparate lot of research still elude the experts. And it's a help when it comes from a prestigious institution, or so it would seem when such research gets a response from a spokesman for the American Heart Association. Dr Richard Stein, from NY University School of Medicine, acknowledged that "this opens up an interesting opportunity for cardiologists to begin to look at the things that one could do to improve psychological wellbeing and to impact global risk".

No-one seems to want to contradict the idea that more positive, optimistic people care better for their health. According to Julia Boehm these positive qualities are associated with lower risk of cardiovascular disease regardless of other factors such as age, body weight, socioeconomic status, even smoking. She claims that "the most optimistic individuals had an approximately 50% reduced risk of experiencing an initial cardiovascular event compared to their less optimistic peers".

More Handy Hints for Stress Reduction

- Siestas: A study from the Harvard School of Public Health in 2007 involving 24,000 subjects found nappers to have a 34% reduced risk of heart disease.

- Breathe deeply: slow abdominal breathing activates the vagus nerve and triggers a relaxation response. Learn more about how simple breathing techniques can lower stress.

- Sing or hum: both release endorphins which reduce stress. Playing and listening to music reduce stress through a variety of mechanisms. Try a drumming workshop.

- Get a massage or a reflexology treatment. Give yourself a foot massage.

- Enjoy the company of your pet, or spend time with someone else's. Pet owners have been shown to have lower cholesterol and triglyceride levels. The presence of a pet has been proven to lower blood pressure and cortisol, as well as increasing happy hormones like oxytocin. Even a fish tank can be therapeutic.

- Laugh. You'll trigger the type of endorphins to help relax your blood vessels.

- Spend time in nature. Become a park walker, a gardener, a beach bum. Research shows even brief bursts of exposure to the natural world lower stress markers such as heart rate, blood pressure and muscle tension. And while you're at it, make sure you go barefoot sometimes. Cardiologist, Stephen Sinatra, regards "grounding" (being in direct contact with the earth) as the most important discovery he has encountered in many years of medical practice.

- Rescue Remedy: Energy medicine? Interestingly it works well for kids and animals (and some human adults if they have an open mind).

- Aromatherapy: lavender baths, frankincense, sandalwood. Research indicates that ylang ylang decreases blood pressure and increases skin temperature. Subjects rated themselves more calm and relaxed than controls. (13)

- Try yoga. Inverse postures, i.e. raising legs above heart, are an example of how yoga may help lower cortisol levels.

- Respirate: medically-approved technology to manage breathing for lowering blood pressure and reducing stress. Can't afford the machine? Try whistling.

- Learn about mindfulness. You could start by reading The Power of Now by Eckhart Tolle or explore some of the many online resources like Dr Rick Hanson's *Just One Minute*. http://justoneminute.net/

- Practice gratitude. Keep a diary of the things you enjoy and the things you appreciate, however small. Note the kindnesses you have received and those you have offered to others.

- Smell the roses. They contain a chemical called linalool, which really can help lower stress. It's that mixture of floral with a touch of spice. You can also get a stress-lowering effect from lavender, mint, lemon, mango, bergamot and many, many more.

It's an exciting challenge that lies ahead in health care. Will it be more about "wellbeing" or "illbeing"? Can we focus more on cultivating our health assets, like optimism, happiness, mindfulness, as well as good food and exercise. Do we need to focus so much on so-called "risk factors" of which there are more every week, but with very little in the way of treatment options. As Kubansky says: "these findings suggest that an emphasis on bolstering psychological strengths rather than simply mitigating psychological deficits may improve cardiovascular health". A good gardener doesn't spend all his time pulling weeds. He mulches, fertilizes, waters and does whatever else he can to encourage the optimal health of his plants. (14)

Chapter 13: Final Thoughts

Now it's time to review your diet and lifestyle with the view of introducing some of the changes we've been discussing. It's an empowering concept to get to the causes of your metabolic problems. Every step you take will help to ensure that your biochemical pathways are working optimally.

You'll now have a better idea about how to balance the types of fat in your diet. You'll want to start eliminating sugar and refined grain products. Understanding the incredible power of natural foods will inspire you to maximize food-derived antioxidants and anti-inflammatory phytochemicals on a daily basis.

The following simple dietary guideline is very similar to that of our ancestors. It will keep us healthier.

Foods to include:

- Meat, lamb, turkey, pork, chicken and organ meats, preferably pasture fed.

- Free range chickens.

- Wild game meats such as venison, kangaroo, boar, buffalo, duck, quail, goose.

- Cold pressed olive oil, unoxidized butter or ghee, coconut oil.

- All seafood including deep sea cold water fish, clams, mussels, oysters, abalone, calamari, squid, roe. Try to get fresh non-polluted varieties.

- Eggs should be from free range chickens and have bright yellow yolks.

- Vegetables should emphasize the non-starchy variety including celery, cucumber, avocados, spinach, broccoli, squash peppers, tomatoes, onion, shallots, garlic, chard and others from the superfoods list.

- Fruits should be of the low GI type. Berries are preferred. Small apples, pears and bananas are fine in moderation for most people.

- Nuts including cashews, pistachios, pecans, almonds, walnuts, macadamia and hazelnuts. They are good sources of essential fatty acids when not consuming seed oils.

- Seeds are also good sources of essential fatty acids and may include sunflower, sesame, pumpkin, pine nuts. Tahini is a useful product.

- Probiotic-containing naturally fermented foods such as plain yoghurt, sauerkraut, kimchi, kefir.

Foods that should be avoided include:

- Refined cereal products such as cakes, biscuits, Danish pastry, scones, pizzas, pasta and other pre-packaged and processed foods containing flour and sugars.
- All confectionary due to high levels of sucrose, fructose and high fructose corn syrup.
- All seed oils which include corn, soya, sunflower, safflower should either be avoided all together or taken in small quantities. Those oils you do use should be cold pressed, fresh and organic, and stored in the refrigerator. Avoid cooking at high temperatures and don't deep fry.
- Trans fats and hydrogenated oils.

Simply keep in mind that foods containing antioxidants and natural anti-inflammatory agents are invariably found in fruits, vegetables, herbs and spices, nuts, legumes and whole grains. Many people have written about "rainbow" foods and it's a good rule of thumb to incorporate as many different coloured foods into the daily diet as possible. Such foods contain the protective phytonutrients we are aiming for, including polyphenolics, flavonoids, carotenoids, anthocyanins, OPCs, catechins, isoflavones and literally thousands of small naturally- occurring molecules. Together with free range sources of animal protein, they contain the major antioxidant vitamins such as vitamins A, C, E, D, K and trace elements such as zinc, manganese, copper and selenium which are part of the antioxidant enzyme system which we synthesize in our body.

A good intake of whole, seasonal, unprocessed foods will help to protect the fatty acids and proteins in the body so that we do not form oxidized fatty acids and other damaging free radicals. If we also cut down on the sugar we get further protection from advanced glycated end products (AGEs) as well as a reduction in the small dense LDL.

Intake of a wide variety of protective phytonutrients will also help ensure that the LDL packages in our blood include antioxidant/anti-inflammatory substances such as quercetin, alpha and beta carotene, coenzyme Q10, lutein/zeaxanthin, astaxanthin, epicatechin, resveratrol, the vitamin E complex and others. These are the substances which protect the LDL from oxidation and forming the more dangerous small, dense LDL which has greater artery uptake and retention and tends to form foam cells, the precursors of plaque.

As for improving the fat balance in the diet, we have pointed out the need to include more omega-3 oils. Remember the balance of omega-6:omega-3 oils in our diet should be closer to 2:1 not 20:1 as found in most 21st century diets. If you need a bit of help to restore this balance, it's not a bad idea to join the rush for omega-3 supplements in health food stores and pharmacies. If you don't want to get these important oils from supplements and prefer a food source, the best is from deep-sea cold-water fish and other cold-water seafood. Unfarmed fish is nutritionally superior. Also be aware of the pollution problem. Through bio-magnification smaller fish are eaten by medium sized fish, which are then eaten by large fish, thus concentrating toxic heavy metals. Some larger fish contain mercury levels that are not acceptable, especially for pregnant women. At the time of writing the fish species most under question is tuna.

As for vegetable oil, a good choice is cold-pressed extra virgin olive oil, which contains all of the original antioxidant/anti-inflammatory compounds. We should stop being afraid of butter, one of the stable of much-maligned saturated fats. As we've discussed, much of the composition of saturated fat, when it's fresh and of good quality, is actually good for your health or at least not bad for you. All things in moderation. Try cooking occasionally with a mixture of butter and olive oil. This gives a wonderful flavour, is very stable and is one of the preferred ways of cooking of the Italians who have a history of low incidence of heart disease. Keep the temperature moderate to low.

Finally, reread the chapter on stress and exercise. Choose your favorite exercise and stress reduction methods and find a way to incorporate them into daily life. Practice them regularly and enjoy.

References

Chapter 1

(1)   Kritchevsk D et al., Effect of cholesterol vehicle in experimental atherosclerosis. Am. J. Physiol., 178, 30–32 (1954).

(2)   Kritchevsky, D & Tepper, SA. Experimental atherosclerosis in rabbits fed cholesterol-free diets: influence of chow components. J. Atheroscler. Res., 8, 357–69 (1968).

(3)   Keys A et al., The diet and 15-year death rate in the seven countries study. Am J Epidemiol 1986;124(6); 903–15.

(4)   Castelli W. Concerning the possibility of a Nutr… Arch Int Med, 1992; 152(7):1371–72.

(5)   http://www.ncbi.nlm.nih.gov/pubmed/7050440/3903734

(6)   http://jama.jamanetwork.com/article.aspx?articleid=182557

(7)   http://www.westonaprice.org/know-your-fats/skinny-on-fats

(8)   http://cista.net/books/Nourishing%20Traditions%20-%20Sally%20Fallon/Nourishing%20Traditions%20-%20Sally%20Fallon.pdf

(9)   Evans AE et al., Autres pays, autres coeurs? Dietary patterns, risk factors and ischaemic heart disease in Belfast and Toulouse. QJM 1995;88(7):469–477.

(10) Lopez-Miranda J. La dieta mediterranea mejora la resistancia a la oxidacion de las lipoproteinas de baja densidad (LDL). Medicina Clinica 115(10):361–65.

(11) Shibata H et al., Nutrition for the Japanese elderly, Nutr Health 1992;8(2-3):165–75.

(12) Franklyn Deborah, "Take a Lesson from the People of Okinawa," Health, September 1996, pp 57–63.

Chapter 2

(1)   http://www.psychiatrictimes.com/mood-disorders/statins-cholesterol-depletion%E2%80%94and-mood-disorders-what%E2%80%99s-link

(2)   Hummel L et al., Serum lipoproteins improve after successful pharmacologica antidepressant treatment; a randomized open-label prospective trial. J Clin Psychiatry 2011; 72(7): 885–91.

(3)   http://evolutionarypsychiatry.blogspot.com.au/2010/12/your-brain-loves-cholesterol-dont-go.html

(4)   Zureik M et al., Serum cholesterol concentration and death from suicide in men; Paris prospective study I BMJ 1996; 313 (7058): 649.

(5)   Valvski M et al., Serum cholesterol levels and suicidal tendencies in psychiatric inpatients. J Clin Psychiatry 1994;55(6) 252–54.

(6)   Golier JA. Low serum cholesterol level and attempted suicide. Am J Psychiatry 1995;152: 419–23.

(7)   Golomb BA. Cholesterol and violence: Is there a connection? Ann Intern Med 1998;128(6): 478–87.

(8)   Virkkune M. Serum cholesterol in antisocial personality Neuropsychobiology 1979; 5(1): 27–30.

(9)   Partonen T et al., Association of low serum total cholesterol with major depression and suicide. Brit l Psychiatry 1999;175: 259–62.

(10)   Ancelin ML et al., Gender and genotype modulation of the association between lipid levels and depressive symptomatology in community-dwelling elderly (the ESPIRIT study). Biol Psychiatry 2010; 68(2): 125–32.

(11)   Morgan RE et al., Plasma cholesterol and depressive symptoms in older men. Lancet 1993;341(1): 75–79.

(12)   Symptoms of Adrenal Gland Deficiency, eHow.com http://www.ehow.com/about_5149995_symptoms-adrenal-gland-deficiency.html#ixzz1X3KX6LZN

Chapter 3

(1)   http://www.ncbi.nlm.nih.gov/pmc/articles/PMC2956535/

(2)   http://www.greenhealthwatch.com/newsstories/newsdirtymedicine/
why-statins-are-bad-idea.html

(3)   Krumholz, HM et al., Lack of association between cholesterol and
coronary heart disease mortality and morbidity and all-cause
mortality in persons older than 70 years JAMA 1994; 272(17),1335–40.

(4)   Weverling-Rijnsberger, AWE. Total cholesterol and risk of mortality
in the oldest old. Lancet 1997; 350: 1119–23.

(5)   Schatz IJ et al., Cholesterol and all cause mortality in elderly people
from the Honolulu Heart Program. Lancet 2001; 358,351–55.

(6)   Kirkby L et al., Lipid-lowering treatment to the end? A review of
observational studies and RCTs on cholesterol and mortality in 80+-
year olds. Age and Ageing. 2010;39(6):674–82.

(7)   Forette B et al., Cholesterol as risk factor for mortality in elderly
women. Lancet 1989; 1:868–70.

(8)   Ulmer H et al., Why Eve is not Adam: prospective follow-up in149650
women and men of cholesterol and other risk factors related to
cardiovascular and all-cause mortality. J Womens Health (Larchmt)
2004; 13(1):41–53.

(9)   Schupf N et al., Relationship between plasma lipids and all-cause
mortality in nondemented elderly. J Am Geriatr Soc 2005; 53: 219–26.

(10)   Onder G et al., Serum cholesterol levels and in-hospital mortality in
the elderly. Am J Med 2003; 115(4): 265–71.

Chapter 4

(1)   http://www.greenhealthwatch.com/newsstories/newsdirtymedicine/
why-statins-are-bad-idea.html

(2)   http://functionaldiagnosticnutrition.com/evidence-mounts-against-
statin-drugs/

(3)   LaRosa JC et al., Intensive lipid lowering with atorvastatin in patients
with stable coronary disease N Engl J Med 2005;352(14):1425–35.

(4)   http://www.ncbi.nlm.nih.gov/pubmed/15755765

(5)   Amarenco P et al., High dose atorvastatin after stroke or transient
ischaemic attack. N Engl J Med 355(6);549–59.

(6)   Kausik K et al., Statins cause all-cause mortality in high-risk primary
prevention. A meta-analysis of 11 randomized controlled trials
involving 65,229 participants. Arch Intern Med 2010;170(12):1024–
31.

(7)   Ghirlanda et al., Evidence of plasma CoQ10-lowering effect of HMG-
CoA reductase inhibitors: a double-blind, placebo-controlled study. J
Clin Pharmacol, 1993; 33(3):226–29.

(8)   Golomb BA & Evans MA. Statin adverse effects: a review of the
literature and evidence for a mitochondrial mechanism. Am J
Cardiovasc Drugs. 2008;8(6):373–418.

(9)   Langsjoen PH et al., Treatment of statin adverse effects with
supplemental coenzyme Q10 and statin drug discontinuatio.n
Biofactors 2005;25(1-4): 147–52.

(10) Vredevoe DL et al., Skin test anergy in advanced heart failure
secondary to either ischemic or idiopathic dilated cardiomyopathy.
Am J Cardiol 1998;82:323–28.

(11) Rauchhaus M et al., The relationship between cholesterol and survival
in patients with chronic heart failure. J Am Coll Cardiol
2003;42(11);1933–40.

(12) Fonarow GC & Horwich TB. Cholesterol and mortality in heart
failure: The bad gone good. J Am Coll Cardiol 42(11) 1941–43.

(13) Horwich TB & Fonarow GC. Statin therapy is associated with
improved survival in ischemic and non-ischemic heart failure. . J Am
Coll Cardiol 43(4) 642–48.

(14) Klotz O et al., Fatty streaks in the intima of arteries. J Path Baceriol
1911; 16(1) 211–20.

Chapter 5

(1)   Klotz O et al., Fatty streaks in the intima of arteries. J Path Baceriol 1911; 16(1) 211–20.

(2)   www.time.com/time/magazine/article/0,9171,843958,00.html

(3)   Circulation http://circ.ahajournals.org/content/108/12/e81.full

(4)   Warnburg J et al., Inflammatory proteins are related to total and abdominal adiposity in a healthy adolescent population: the AVENA Study. Am J Clin Nutr 2006; 84:505–12.

(5)   Fontana L et al., Long-term calorie restriction is highly effective in reducing the risk for atherosclerosis in humans. PNAS 2004;101(17): 6659–63.

(6)   http://thefastdiet.co.uk/

Chapter 6

(1)   Dr W Davis, Life Extension. 2005 Mar; 11(3):114–24.

(2)   Lamarche B et al., The small dense LDL phenotype and the risk of coronary heart disease. Epidemiology, patho-physiology and therapeutic aspects. Diabetes Metab. 1999; 25, 199–211.

(3)   Esterbauer H et al., Effect of antioxidants on oxidative modification of LDL. Ann Med. 1991; 23(5):573–81.

(4)   www.drlam.com/opinion/Lp(a).asp

(5)   Singh RB & Niaz MA. Serum concentration of lipoprotein(a) decreases on treatment with hydrosoluble coenzyme Q10 in patients with coronary artery disease: discovery of a new role. Int J Cardiol 1999 68(1): 23–29.

(6)   Austin MA et al., Low-density lipoprotein subclass patterns and risk of myocardial infarction. JAMA 1988; 260(13), 1917–21.

(7)   Finn R. Saturated fat may slow atherosclerosis in women. Cardiovascular Medicine. Internal Medicine News, June 15, 2004.

(8)   Mikhailidis DP et al., HDL-cholesterol and the treatment of coronary heart disease: contrasting effects of atorvastatin and simvastatin. Curr Med Res Opin. 2000; 16(2) 139–46.

(9)   Nichols GA et al., Change in high-density lipoprotein cholesterol and risk of subsequent hospitalization for coronary artery disease or stroke among patients with type 2 diabetes mellitus. Am J Cardiol 2011;108(8):1124–28.

(10) Ashen MD et al., Clinical practice. Low HDL levels. N Engl J Med 2005; 353: 1252–60.

(11) Rader DJ. Cholesterol Efflux Capacity, High-Density Lipoprotein Function, and Atherosclerosis, N Eng J Med 2011; 364:127–35.

(12) Ferretti G et al., HDL-paraoxonase and membrane lipid peroxidation: A comparison between healthy and obese subjects. Obesity.18(6): 1072–84.

Chapter 7

(1) Toborek M et al., Unsaturated fatty acids selectively induce an inflammatory environment in human endothelial cells. Am J Clin Nutr 2002; 75:119–25.

(2) Perez RV. Dietary immunoregulation of trqnsfusion-induced immunosuppression. Transplanttion 1988 45(3): 614–17.

(3) http://www.heartfoundation.org.au/healthy-eating/fats/Pages/butter-margarine.aspx

(4) Willett W et al., Trans fatty acids: Are the effects only marginal? Circulation 1994; 84;(5):722–24.

(5) Simopoulos AP. The importance of the ratio of omega-6/omega-3 essential fatty acids. Biomed Pharmacother 2002;56(8):365–79.

(6) Frasure-Smith N et al., Major depression is associated with lower omega-3 fatty acid levels in patients with recent acute coronary syndromes. Biol Psych 2004; 55(9) 891–96.

(7) http://customers.hbci.com/~wenonah/new/canola.htm

(8) Christakis G et al., The anti-coronary club. A dietary approach to the prevention of coronary heart disease-a seven-year report. Am J Pub Health Nation Health 1966; 56(2): 299–314.

(9) http://www.health-report.co.uk/saturated_fats_health_benefits.htm

(10) Burlingame B et al., Fats and Fatty Acids in Human Nutrition. Ann Nutr Metab. 2009; 55, 5–7.

(11) Siri-Tarino PW, Sun Q, Hu FB & Krauss RM. Meta-analysis of prospective cohort studies evaluating the association of saturated fat with cardiovascular disease. Am J Clin Nutr. 2010 Mar;91(3):535–46.

(12) Astrup A et al., The role of reducing intakes of saturated fat in the prevention of cardiovascular disease; where does the evidence stand in 2010. Am J Clin Nutr 2011; 93(4): 684–88.

(13) Micha R & Mozaffarian D. Saturated fat and cardiometabolic risk factors, coronary heart disease, stroke and diabetes: a fresh look at the evidence. Lipids 2010; 45(10): 893–905.

(14) Gillman MW et al., Inverse Association of Dietary Fat with Development of Ischemic Stroke in Men. JAMA 1997; 278 (24): 2145–2150.

(15) Mensink RP et al., Effects of dietary fatty acids and carbohydrates on the ratio of serum total to HDL cholesterol and on serum lipids and apolipoproteins: a meta-analysis of 60 controlled trials. Am J Clin Nutr 2003;77:1146–1155.

(16) French MA et al., Cholesterolaemic effect of palmitic acid in relation to other dietary fatty acids. Asia Pacific J Clin Nutr 2002;11 suppl s7 S401–S407.

(17) Newens KJ et al., DHA-rich fish oil reverses the detrimental effects of saturated fatty acids on postprandial vascular reactivity. Am J Clin Nutr 2011; 94:742–48.

(18) Dhiman TR et al., Conjugated linoleic acid content of milk from cows fed different diets. J Dairy Sci 1999 Oct; 82(10):2146–56.

(19) Nicolosi RJ et al., Dietary conjugated linoleic acid reduces plasma lipoproteins and early aortic atherosclerosis in hypercholesterolemic hamsters. Artery 1997; 22(5):266–77.

(20) Simopoulos A. Omega-3 fatty acids in health and disease and in growth and development. Am J Clin Nutr 1991, 54:438–63.

(21) Bell SJ et al., Health implications of milk containing beta casein with the A2 genetic variant. Crit Rev Food Sci Nutr 2006; 46(1):93–100.

(22) Tailford KA et al., A casein variant in cow's milk is atherogenic. Atherosclerosis 2003; 170(1):13–19.

(23) Hu FB et al., A prospective study of egg consumption and risk of cardiovascular disease in men and women. JAMA 1999; 281 (15):1387–1394.

(24) https://www.sciencenews.org/blog/food-thought/reevaluating-eggs-cholesterol-risks

(25) Chowdhury R et al., Association of dietary, circulating, and supplementary fatty acids with coronary risk: A systematic review and meta-analysis. Ann Intern med 2014;160(6):398–406.

Chapter 8

(1)   http://www.ncbi.nlm.nih.gov/pmc/articles/PMC3258689/

(2)   Zhang L et al., Proteomic analysis of fructose-induced fatty liver in hamsters. Metabolism.2008;57(8): 1115–24.

(3)   Seneff S. Is the metabolic syndrome caused by a high fructose, and relatively low fat, low cholesterol diet? Arch Med Sci 2011; 7(1): 8–20.

(4)   Aeberli I et al., Fructose intake is a predictor of LDL particle size in overweight schoolchildren. Am J Clin Nutr 2007; 86(4):1174–1178.

(5)   Gaziano JM et al., Fasting triglycerides, high-density lipoprotein, and risk of myocardial infarction. Circulation 1997; 96:2520–2525.

(6)   Stanhope KL et al., Consumption of fructose and high fructose corn syrup increase postprandial tiglycerides, LDL-cholesterol, and apolipoprotein-B in young men and women. Journal of Clinical Endocrinology & Metabolism, 2011.

(7)   Johnson RJ et al., Potential role of sugar (fructose) in the epidemic of hypertension, obesity and the metabolic syndrome, diabetes, kidney disease and cardiovascular disease. Am J Clin Nutr 2007; 86: 899–906.

Chapter 9

(1)   Aviram M et al., Pomegranate juice consumption, http://www.ncbi.nlm.nih.gov/pubmed/15158307

(2)   Chai SC et al., Comparative effects of dried plum: impact on cardiovascular disease risk factors in postmenopausal women. J Acad Nutr Diet 2012;112(8): 1158–68.

Chapter 11

(1)   Grey KF et al., Plasma levels of antioxidant vitamins in relation to ischemic heart disease and cancer. Am J Clin Nutr 1987;45:1368–77.

(2)   Aggarwal BB et al., Tocotrienols, the vitamin E of the 21st Century: Its potential against cancer and other chronic diseases. Biochem Pharmacol 2010; 80(11) 1613–1631.

(3)   Jordan KG. What's wrong with vitamin E? Life Extension May 2002.

(4)   Mollace V et al., Hypolipemic and hypoglycaemic activity of bergamot polyphenols: From animal models to human studies, Fitoterapia (2011) 82;309–316.

(5)   Janikula M. Policosanol: a new treatment for cardiovascular disease? Alt Med Rev 2002;7(3)203–217.

(6)   Braun L. Policosanol: sugarcane wax wanes in trials. J Coml. Med. 2009, 8(4) 46–47.

(7)   Soni KB & Kuttan R. Effect of oral curcumin administration on serum peroxides and cholesterol levels in human volunteers. Indian J Physiol Pharmacol 36(4) 273–75 (1992).

(8)   Peschel D et al., Curcumin induces changes in expression of genes involved in cholesterol homeostasis. J Nutr Biochem 2007;18(2): 113–19.

(9)   Dou X et al., Curcumin up-regulates LDL receptor expression via the sterol regulatory element pathway in HepG2 cells. Planta Med. 2008 Sep;74(11):1374–79.

(10) Borek, C. Health and Anti-Aging Benefits of Aged Garlic Extract 288, 72–73 (2007).

(11) Satyavati GV, A promising hypolipidaemic agent from gum guggal (Commiphora Wightii). Econ Med Plant Res 1991; 5: 47–82.

(12) Fukushima M et al., Cholesterol-lowering effects of maitake (Grifola frondosa) fiber, shiitake (Lentinus edodes) fiber, and enokitake (Flammulina velutipes) fiber in rats. Exp Biol Med (Maywood). 2001; 226(8):758–65.

(13) Bobek P et al., Dietary oyster mushroom (Pleurotus ostreatus) accelerates plasma cholesterol turnover in hypercholesterolaemic rat. Physiol Res 1995; 44(5):287–91.

(14) Cooke JP & Zimmer J. The Cardiovascular Cure: Your Self-Defense Against Heart Attack and Stroke. Random House. 2002.

Chapter 12

(1)   Myers J, Circulation. 2003;107:e2–e3.

(2)   Myers J et al., Exercise capacity and mortality among men referred for exercise testing. N Engl J Med.2002;346:793–801.

(3)   American College of Sports Medicine. Guidelines for Exercise Testing and Prescription, 6th ed. Baltimore, Md: Lippincott Williams & Wilkins; 2000.

(4)   Australian Heart Foundation—Active Living www.heartfoundation.com.au

(5)   Houmard JA et al., Effects of exercise training on the chemical composition of plasma LDL. Arterioscler Thromb.1994; 14(3):325–30.

(6)   Williams PT et al., Lipoprotein subfractions of runners and sedentary men. Metabolism. 1986;35(1):45.

(7)   Kazuhiko K et al., The correlation between small dense LDL and reactive metabolites in a physical activity intervention in hyperlipidemic subjects J Clin Med Res; 4(3):161–166.

(8)   Mikus CR et al., Simvastatin impairs exercise training adaptations. J Am Coll, Cardiol. 2013;62(8):709–14.

(9)   Killewich LA et al., Exercise enhances endogenous fibrinolysis in peripheral arterial disease. J Vasc Surg. 2004; 40(4):741.

(10) Lynch James J. The Language of the Heart. The Human Body in Dialogue. Basic Books NY 1938.

(11) Benson Herbert, The Relaxation Response. HarperTorch NY 2000.

(12) http://virginialee.org/wordpress/?p=151

(13) Hongratanaworakit T et al., Relaxing effect of ylang ylang oil on humans after transdermal absorption. Phytother Res.2006;20(9):758–63.

(14) Boehm J & Kubzansky L. The Heart's Content: The association between positive psychological well-being and cardiovascular health. Psych Bull. 2012;138(4): 655–691.

www.ingramcontent.com/pod-product-compliance
Lightning Source LLC
Chambersburg PA
CBHW041309210326
41599CB00003B/36